쉬운 영어로 과학논문 쓰는 법

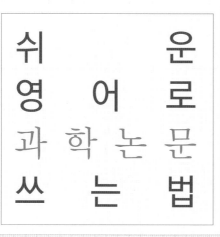

쉬운 영어로 과학논문 쓰는 법

ANNE E. GREENE 지음

안성민 옮김

군자출판사

목차

CONTENTS

Welcome to the Korean translation of *Writing Science in Plain English*. Learning a difficult language like English is hard. Learning to write complex science in English is harder still. The fact that you are reading this preface means that you are willing to go one step further – to evaluate your scientific writing and try to improve it. Congratulations!

I teach scientific writing to senior undergraduates and graduate students. Many believe that when they write science, they must be formal, abstract, and impersonal. They copy what they read in the scientific literature and use long complicated words, abstract terms, and passive verbs. Their writing is wordy, convoluted, and hard to understand.

One of my goals is to convince these students that a lot of what they read in the literature is badly written. It is a poor model for their own writing. While there are certainly good scientific writers, many others fail to give readers what they need to understand complex ideas. What readers need from writers is what this book is all about. For instance, our readers need stories about concrete things doing some kind of action. They need short words that are easy to understand, and they need certain kinds of information in the right places in paragraphs and sentences.

This information surprises many of my students and may surprise you too. It is natural to use the scientific literature as a model and take phrases and words from it to express your ideas. This book will help you re-think those tendencies and write in a different way with different goals. With practice, you may no longer feel the need to impress or to conform but rather to write clearly, in simpler English, so that your colleagues and even a broader audience can understand you easily.

I am very fortunate to have the support of my publication team at the University of Chicago Press, my editors at The University of Montana, and my family. I am deeply grateful to Sung-Min Ahn who spearheaded this project and did the hard work of translating the text. It was his determination to see clearer scientific writing in English that made this book possible.

Anne Greene
July 2015

역자 서문

이외수의 "글쓰기의 공중부양"이란 책을 보고 너털 웃음을 지었다. 글쓰기를 공중
부양할 수 있다면 얼마나 좋을까? 물론 글쓰기가 공중부양만큼이나 어렵다는 의미가
숨어있으리라.

역자도 글쓰기에 적지않은 공을 들였다. 첫째는 글재주가 없고, 둘째는 글쓰기를
제대로 배워본 적이 없어서다. 영어가 좀 낫다는 죄로 의과대학 시절에는 영문 초록
이나 논문 고쳐쓰는 일에 적지 않게 불려다녔다. 논문작성법을 배워보지도 못하고 간
신히 고쳐쓰면서 영어논문 쓰는 법을 제대로 공부해보자고 결심했고 급기야는 Mimi
Zeiger가 집필한 "Essentials of Writing Biomedical Papers[1]"를 2년 간에 걸쳐 번역하기
에 이르렀다. 이 책은 최대 12주 동안의 영어논문 교육코스의 교재로 사용되며 상세
한 설명과 예문이 곁들어진 바이블이다. 번역하면서 많은 것을 배웠고 그 경험은 멜
번대학에서 박사과정을 밟으면서 10만 단어에 이르는 박사학위 논문을 작성하는데
큰 도움이 되었다.

그 후에도 논문작성이나 글쓰기와 관련한 책을 이십 권 남짓 보았지만 별다른 소
득은 없었고 더욱이 영어논문에 관한 또 다른 책을 번역해보고자 하는 생각은 해보
지 않았다.

이 책을 알게된 것은 호기심에서다. 과학논문을 쉬운 영어로 쓸 수 있다니. 이 책
의 원제목인 "Writing science in plain English"는 "글쓰기의 공중부양" 만큼이나 매력
적으로 들렸다. 유명 과학저널 에디터들의 추천이 잇따랐다. 저자 본인도 과학자이자

---

1. Mini Zeiger의 생의학 영어논문작성법 2판 / 안성민 역 / 군자출판사

과학저널의 에디터다. 어떤 책일까? 우선은 책이 아주 얇았다. 분량은 Mimi Zeiger 책의 1/10 정도. 별 생각없이 책장을 처음 넘긴 다음 앉은 자리에서 끝까지 다 읽게되었고, 공중부양을 경험했다. 더 완전하게 내 것으로 만들고 싶어서 일주일에 걸쳐 번역을 마무리했다.

영어가 모국어가 아닌 대부분의 한국 과학자에게는 이 책의 울림이 더욱 크리라 생각된다. 학생시절 틈틈히 모아 발췌해두었던 문장들 대부분이 현학적이고, 모호하며, 피해야 할 문장이라는 점을 이 책을 통해 깨달았다. 좋은 과학논문은 정말 쉬운 문장으로 씌여졌다는 점을 확인했다. 우리도 알고 있지 않은가? 정말 깊게 이해하고 있는 주제는 누구에게라도 쉽게 설명할 수 있다는 사실을. 이 책을 통해 여러분도 글쓰기의 공중부양을 경험하게 되리라 확신한다. 쉽게 쓰자. 쉬운 언어로 깊이 있는 연구를 자신있게 드러내자. 모국어가 아닌 언어를 가지고 더 어려운 단어, 더 어려운 문장으로 논문을 쓰고자 고심하는 연구자에게 이 책이 시원한 소나기가 되었으면 한다.

마지막으로, 번역문의 교정에 도움을 준 연구소의 김덕훈, 신지연, 오승준, 이선영에게 감사의 말을 전한다.

안성민

About the Author : Anne Greene
July 2015

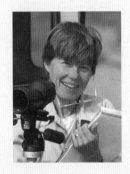

I received my Bachelor of Science and Master of Science degrees from Dalhousie University in Halifax, Nova Scotia, Canada. While there, I conducted research on marine invertebrates and Atlantic seabirds off the coasts of Nova Scotia and Newfoundland. Later, I worked for the Canadian Wildlife Service studying seabirds at a colony on Prince Leopold Island in the Eastern Canadian Arctic.

I have always loved writing and literature and am particularly interested in writing science for a broad audience. I have written for numerous natural history organizations, museums, magazines, and newspapers. I have been a writing tutor for elementary, middle school, and high school students for years and worked at the Writing Center at The University of Montana (UM) helping undergraduate and graduate students with their scientific writing. I have taught an honors course in scientific writing at UM for over a decade and enjoy giving writing workshops to students of all ages and scientific disciplines.

역자: 안성민 MD-PhD
2015년 7월

학력

BSc in Biochemistry and Molecular Biology, the University of Queensland
MD, 아주대학교 의과대학
PhD, Ludwig Institute for Cancer Research, the University of Melbourne,
with emphasis on genomics and proteomics

경력

가천대 기초의학부 분자의학과 조교수 / 가천대 길병원 중개의학과 조교수
가천대 기초의학부 분자의학과 부교수 / 가천대 길병원 중개의학과 부교수
서울아산병원 종양내과/의생명정보학과 촉탁임상교수(현)
서울아산병원 아산생명과학연구원 연구기획관리실 부실장(현)
서울아산병원 암병원 암연구기획 책임교수(현)

수상경력

21세기를 이끌 우수인재상(대통령상) / Australia-Asia Awards / 연강학술상

역서

의생명정보학 기법 Jules J. Berman 저/ 안성민 등 역 허원미디어 2014
At the Bench Kathy Barker 저/ 안성민, 박상진, 홍성호 공역 월드사이언스 2008
Mimi Zeiger의 생의학 영어논문 작성법 2판 Mimi Zeiger저/안성민 역 군자출판사 2005
세포의 반란 로버트 와인버그 저/조혜성, 안성민 공역 사이언스북스 2005
생물학 실험을 위한 수학 Dany Adanms 저/안성민 등 역 월드사이언스 2005

대표논문

주저자로 Hepatology, Genome Research, Oncogene 등의 저널에 다수의 논문 발표

제1장

쉬운 영어로 논문을 써야하는 이유

"논문 읽는게 힘들지 않나요?" 과학논문작성법 강의 첫 시간에 이런 질문을 던져 본다. 생물학 석사 학생들은 고개를 끄덕인다. 과학논문을 읽는 것이 어렵다는데 동의하는 것이다. 이유를 물으면 이런 답변이 나온다. "논문 읽으면 졸려요", "서너 번 읽어야 무슨 말인지 알 수 있어요", "논문을 읽다보면 제가 바보처럼 느껴져요." 지적이고 정열적인 학생들이 과학논문 읽는 일을 왜 힘들어할까? 이유는 논문 대다수의 글쓰기 수준이 형편없기 때문이다.

학부 학생이라면 숙제로 받은 논문을 읽을 때 비슷한 경험을 할 것이다. 석박사 학생이나 박사후 연구원, 책임연구자라면 비슷한 불평을 학생에게서 듣고 있거나 이런 생각을 직접 해본 적이 있을 것이다.

실제로 많은 저널 에디터와 관록 있는 과학자들이 불명료한 글쓰기를 심각한 문제로 받아들이고 있다. 과학 에디터 협회의 전임 회장이었던 피터 우드포드(Peter Woodford)는 과학저널의 논문에서 볼 수 있는 글쓰기 수준을 끔찍하다고 표현했다.[1] *Nature*의 시니어 에디터인 레슬리 세이지(Leslie Sage)는 다음과 같이 말했다. "씁쓸하기는 하지만 *Nature*에 투고되는 '엉터리' 논문의 상당수가 글쓰기의 관점에서만 보자면 진짜배기 논문의 상당수보다 수준이 높다."[2] *Integrative and Comparative Biology*의 에디터인 해롤드 히트월(Harold Heatwole)의 결론은 다음과 같다. "현재 과학저널의 글쓰기 표준은 빈약한 문법과 부정확한 커뮤니케이션 관점 모두에서 전 시대에 거쳐 가장 낮은 수준에 이르렀다."[3] 이 주제에 관해 기고한 고참 과학자의 대부분은 과학논문이 "불필요하게 무미건조하며, 읽기 어렵고, 애매모호하다는"[4] 데이비드 포러시(David Porush)의 의견에 뜻을 같이한다. 이들은 과학자가 좀 더 명료하고 직접적이며 정확하게[5-8], 즉 안토니 윌슨(Anthony wilson)이 말한 "쉽고 단순한 영어로"[9] 논문을 써야 한다고 주장한다.

양적으로는 폭발적으로 증가하고 있는 과학논문이 질적으로는 개선되지 않고 있다.[10] 대기과학 분야의 22개의 저널을 조사한 바에 의하면 논문 명료성 지표는 정체중이거나 하락하고 있었다.[11] 2011년 12월에는 *Science Signaling*의 총괄 에디터가 많은 논문 원고의 생물정보학 분석 결과가 "모호하고 얽혀있으며, 불필요한 전문용어가 남용되고 내용 파악이 불가능하다"고 언급한 바 있다.[12] 과학논문의 글쓰기 수준이 전반적으로 빈약하다고 문제될 것이 있을까? 글쓰기 수준이 낮으면 서로 다른 분야 간에 아이디어의 자유로운 흐름이 어려워진다. 과학은 점점 세분화되고 있는데 과학논문의 글이 복잡해지면 전문가들이 서로 다른 분야를 이해하기 어렵다.[13] 과거에는 서로 다른 분야의 교잡을 통해 과학이 진보해왔다. 글쓰기의 수준이 낮으면 한 분야에서 이루어진 발견을 다른 분야에 적용하기가 더 어려워진다.[11, 14] 최근 한 과학자는 불명료한 글쓰기가 과학적 프로세스 자체를 방해한다고 주장한 바 있다.[12]

수준이 낮은 글쓰기는 과학에 대한 대중의 이해도를 낮추고 과학자와 대중의 커뮤니케이션을 어렵게 한다.[4, 9, 15-17] 이렇게 심각한 문제를 해결하기 위해서는 과학에 이해심 깊은 시민과 법률제정가들이 모종의 결단을 마련할 필요가 있다.[18] "국민과 언론을 위한 퓨 연구센터"가 최근 수행한 여론조사에 의하면 85%의 과학자가 과학에 관한 대중의 무관심을 심각한 문제로 꼽았다. 조사에 응한 미국인의 50% 가량이 인간 활동이 글로벌 기후 변화를 일으키는 원인이라는 사실에 동의하지 않았으며 1/3 가량은 진화를 믿지 않았다.[19] 이러한 균열을 메꾸기 위해서 미국과학진흥협회 회장인 피터 아그레(Peter Agre)는 "모든 과학자와 공학자가 자신의 연구를 대중에게 유익할 뿐만 아니라 대중이 이해할 수 있도록 만들어야 한다고" 주장했다.[18]

젊은 과학자가 우리의 가장 큰 희망일지 모른다. 비과학적 미국(*Unscientific America*)이라는 저서에서 저자인 크리스 무니(Chris Mooney)와 쉐릴 커쉔바움(Sheril Kirshenbaum)은 과학자와 비과학자 간에 존재하는 커다란 소통의 장벽을 묘사하고 있으며 더 효과적으로 소통할 수 있는 르네상스형 과학자를 길러냄으로써 이를 개선할 수 있다고 주장한다.[20] 미국과학진흥협회의 CEO이자 *Science*지의 발행인인 앨런 레쉬너(Alan Leshner)는 젊은 과학자가 "대중 커뮤니케이션" 교육을 받아야 하며, 자신의 연구를 더 많은 청중과 공유하는 과학자를 보상해야 한다

고 믿는다.[21]

과학계의 빈약한 글쓰기 수준은 젊은 과학자에게 나쁜 선례를 제공한다. 과학의 특정 분야에 새로 진입한 신참은 해당 분야 저널의 글쓰기 스타일을 모방한다. 이런 모방은 분야에 상관없이 흔한 일이지만 동시에 빈약한 글쓰기 수준을 지속시킨다.[4, 8, 22] 관록 있는 과학자도 글쓰기 스타일은 지도교수의 영향을 받으며 문제는 지도교수의 대부분이 명료한 글쓰기 교육 또는 명료하게 글쓰기를 가르치는 교육을 받지 못했다는 점이다.[7, 17] 그렇기 때문에 학생이 논문을 들고 갔을 때 지도교수로부터 받는 피드백은 천차만별이다.

좋은 소식은 조셉 윌리엄스(Joseph Wiliams)가 본인의 저서인 "*Style: Toward Clarity and Grace*"[22]에서 전문 작가를 위해 제시한 몇 가지 원칙을 적용함으로써 여러분도 과학논문을 쉬운 영어로 작성할 수 있다는 사실이다. 이 원칙들은 독자가 복잡하고 생소한 정보를 읽을 때 무엇을 찾는지에 관한 언어학적 이론에 기초하고 있다. 원칙 목록은 놀랄 만큼 단순하다: 1) 독자는 주인공과 액션이 있는 스토리, 2) 주어 근처에 위치한 강력한 동사, 3) 문장 앞부분에서는 오래된 정보, 4) 뒷부분에서는 새로운 정보, 5) 문단과 글 전체의 예측 가능한 위치에서 특별한 종류의 정보를 찾는다.

윌리엄스의 원칙 목록과 이들의 언어학적 역사가 이 책의 중심을 이룬다. 과학적 글쓰기에 관한 다른 많은 저서는 과학자가 쓸 **내용**에 초점을 맞춘다. 즉, 박사논문이나 연구계획서, 연구논문, 리뷰논문을 어떻게 준비해야 하는지를 설명한다. 그런 종류의 많은 저서에 데이터 정리 및 포맷, 참고문헌 인용스타일에 관한 지침이 포함되어 있다. 어떤 경우에는 구두발표 및 포스터 준비에 관한 내용이 포함되기도 한다.[5, 8, 23, 24] 이런 저서들은 과학논문이 이해하기 어려운 **이유**와 이를 개선할 수 있는 **방법**에 초점을 맞추고 있지 않다.

이 책은 명료하고 이해하기 쉬운 논문 작성을 위해 과학자가 초점을 맞추어야 할 일에 관한 정보를 제공한다. 이 책이 설명하는 원칙은 과학 분야 글쓰기의 모든 것(연구 노트, 연구비 계획서, 연구 논문 심지어 신문 기사)의 수준을 높여줄 것이다. 글쓰기의 어떤 단계에서 이러한 원칙을 사용할 지는 여러분에게 달려있다. 첫 초고를 교정할 때 사용할 수도 있고, 능숙해진 다음에는 글을 써나가면서 적용할 수도 있다. 이 점만 기억하면 된다. 글을 쓸 때는 특정 단계에서 글을 교정함으로써 여러분의 글이 독자가 여러분을 이해하기 위해 필요한 요소를 제공할 수 있게 해야 한다.

글쓰기에 앞서서 글의 독자와 사용역, 어조를 정할 필요가 있다. 이 주제는 2장에서 다루어진다. 나머지 장에서는 과학논문에서 발췌된 좋은 실례, 나쁜 실례에 기초해서 글쓰기의 원칙이 설명된다. 각 원칙을 이해한 뒤에는 각 장 말미의 연습문제를 이용해서 해당 원칙을 연습해볼 수 있다. 그런 다음 여러분의 결과를 부록 2에 있는 해답과 비교해보라.

이 책에는 흔히 사용되는 문법용어가 몇 가지 사용된다. 용어의 의미를 잘 모르거나 문법을 리뷰하고 싶다면 부록 1을 참조하라. 이 책에 등장하는 문법용어를 이해하는 일은 중요하다. 글쓰기의 원칙이 작동하는 방법을 설명할 때 문법용어가 사용되며 다른 한편으로는 이런 문법용어가 글쓰기의 원칙을 적용하는 일에 도움이 된다.

과학 분야 글쓰기와 관련된 많은 문제는 분야와 수준에 상관없이 보편적이다. 따라서 이 책이 제시하는 원칙은 지질학자, 화학자, 물리학자, 생물학자, 사회과학자이건, 대학 신입생, 졸업반, 석박사 학생, 박사 후 연구원, 교수이건 간에 상관없이 큰 도움이 될 것이다.

물론, 과학논문의 가치는 글쓰기의 스타일만큼이나 그 속에 담겨있는 내용에 좌우된다. 여러분이 설명하고자 하는 과학적 질문과 가설, 실험 디자인과 해석은 마찬가지로 중요하다. 하지만, 이렇게 중요한 내용을 독자와 분명하게 소통할 수 없다면 무슨 가치가 있겠는가?

=== REFERENCE ===

1. Woodford, F. P. Sounder thinking through clearer writing. *Science* **156**, 743–745 (1967).
2. Sage, L. in *Astronomy Communication* (eds Heck, A. & Madsen, C.) 221–225 (Kluwer Academic Publishers, 2003).
3. Heatwole, H. A plea for scholarly writing. *Integr. Comp. Biol.* **48**, 159–163 (2008).
4. Porush, D. *A Short Guide to Writing about Science* (Longman, 1995).
5. Ebel, H. F., Bliefert, C. & Russey, W. E. *The Art of Scientific Writing: From Student Reports to Professional Publications in Chemistry and Related Fields* (Wiley-VCH, 1987).
6. O'Connor, M. *Writing Successfully in Science* (HarperCollins, 1991).
7. Alley, M. *The Craft of Scientific Writing* 3rd edn (Springer, 1996).
8. Schultz, D. M. *Eloquent Science: A Practical Guide to Becoming a Better Writer, Speaker, and Atmospheric Scientist* (The American Meteorological Society, 2009).

9. Wilson, A. *Handbook of Science Communication* (Institute of Physics Publishing, 1998).

10. Wells, W. A. Me write pretty one day: How to write a good scientific paper. *J. Cell Biol.* **165**, 757–58 (2004).

11. Geerts, B. Trends in atmospheric science journals: A reader's perspective. *Bull. Am. Meteorol. Soc.* **80**, 639–51 (1999).

12. Yaffe, M. B. The complex art of telling it simply. *Sci. Signal.* **4**, doi: 10.1126 / scisignal.2002710 (2011).

13. Gould, S. J. Take another look. *Science* **286**, 899 (1999).

14. Sand- Jensen, K. How to write consistently boring scientifi c literature. *Oikos* **116**, 723–27 (2007).

15. White, F. D. *Communicating Technology: Dynamic Processes and Models for Writers* (HarperCollins, 1996).

16. Sabloff, J. A. Distinguished lecture in archeology: Communication and the future of American archaeology. *Am. Anthropol.* **100**, 869–75 (1999).

17. Barrass, R. *Scientists Must Write* 2nd edn (Routledge, 2002).

18. Lempinen, E. W. (ed) Science leaders urge new effort to strengthen bonds with public. *Science* **327**, 1591 (2010).

19. Pew Research Center for the People and the Press. *Scientific Achievements Less Prominent Than a Decade Ago: Public Praises Science; Scientists Fault Public, Media.* Available at http:// www.people-press.org/ reports/ pdf/ 528.pdf (2009).

20. Mooney, C. & Kirshenbaum, S. *Unscientific America: How Scientific Illiteracy Threatens Our Future* (Basic Books, 2009).

21. Leshner, A. I. Outreach training needed. *Science* **315**, 161 (2007).

22. Williams, J. M. *Style: Toward Clarity and Grace* 5th edn (Univ. Chicago Press, 1995).

23. Hofmann, A. H. *Scientific Writing and Communication: Papers, Proposals, and Presentations* (Oxford Univ. Press, 2010).

24. Pechenik, J. A. *A Short Guide to Writing about Biology* 7th edn (Longman, 2010).

제2장
글쓰기에 앞서서

미리 계획하는 일은 대개 유익하다. 특별히 글쓰기에 있어서는 미리 계획하는 것이 성공과 실패를 좌우할 수 있다. 글쓰기에 앞서서 누구를 위해서 쓰는 것이며, 얼마나 격식을 갖추어야 하는지, 원하는 스타일은 무엇인지 결정하라. 그러면 글을 명료하고 흥미롭게 만드는 데 도움이 될 것이다. 과학자들은 때로 무미건조하고 추상적이며 변화가 없는 스타일을 선호하지만 글쓰기에 앞서서 독자와 사용역, 스타일을 고려함으로써 더 좋은 결과를 얻을 수 있다.

| 독자

가장 중요한 첫 번째 단계는 독자를 그려보는 것이다. 누가 여러분의 보고서, 연구논문, 박사논문 또는 텍스트북을 읽을 것인가? 독자에는 가족과 친구, 해당 분야에 흥미가 있는 비과학자 또는 여러분의 전문분야 안팎의 과학자가 포함될 수 있다. 대부분의 경우, 독자의 일부는 해당 주제에 관해 여러분보다 지식이 적을 것이며 따라서 그들의 입장에 설 필요가 있다. 그런 독자들은 여러분을 이해하기 원하지만, **지식이 부족하다**. 여러분의 글을 가능한 명료하게 만들어서 그런 독자를 도우라. 독자가 불분명하다면 보수적으로 해당 주제에 대해 가장 적게 아는 독자층을 대상으로 쓰라. 그렇게 하면, 누구에게도 혼란을 주지 않을 것이며 더 많은 독자에게 나아갈 수 있다.

학생의 경우 독자는 한 명, 즉 지도교수일 것이다. 하지만, 현실 세계에서 여러분은 대단히 다양한 독자층을 위해 글을 쓰게 되며 글쓰기의 성공은 독자 각각과 명료하게 소통할 수 있는지 여부에 좌우되는 경우가 많다. 그러므로 연구논문이나 실험 리포트를 작성할 때 더 넓은 독자층(즉 여러분보다 해당 주제에 관해 잘 모르는)을 상정하고 이들을 대상으로 글을 쓰라. 여러분의 주제에 관해 명료하고 단순하게 글을 쓴다면 지도교수에게 여러분이 그 주제를 이해하고 있다는 점을 보여줄 수 있다.

| 사용역(Register)

사용역은 글이 구어체와 문어체 사이의 어느 지점에 위치하는지 설명해준다 (즉, 얼마나 격식을 차렸는지). 글은 격식을 차릴수록 이해하기 어려우며, 해당 주제를 잘 알지 못하는 독자의 경우 더욱 그렇다. 다음에 등장하는 예제들은 (하나를 제외하고) 고슴도치의 교미 행태라는 유사한 주제를 설명하고 있지만 과학 글쓰기에 사용되는 네 가지 서로 다른 사용역이 사용됐다(구어적; informal, 대중적; popular, 관습적; conventional, 추상적; abstract).[1]

1. 구어적 사용역(INFORMAL REGISTER)

Have you ever wondered, "How the heck do porcupines manage to mate with all those spines everywhere?" Well, the answer to that question is pretty hard to figure out because porcupines are hard to see at the best of times, but it's almost impossible when they're courting. It turns out that the whole affair is up to the woman. When she is ready to become pregnant, she produces a very strong odor that can drive the male porcupine crazy!

우리는 가족이나 친구에게 구어적 사용역을 사용하곤 한다. 구어적 사용역은 회화체이며 감정이 섞이는 경우도 있다. 구어적 사용역은 작가와 독자가 서로 친근하다는 가정 위에 사용되며 좋은 스토리를 엮을 수 있다. 위의 예에서는 "how the heck"이나 "the whole affair is up to the woman"과 같은 구문이 해당 글을 과학적 목적에는 부적합하게 만든다. 하지만, 어떤 경우에는 구어적 사용역을 약간 첨가함으로써 영혼과 열정을 불어넣을 수 있다. 학부생에게 보내는 편지에서 발췌된 아래의 글은 위스콘신 대학의 학부생을 위한 연구 인턴십 프로그램의 지도교수들이 쓴 것이다.

Thank you for your interest in our National Science Foundation Ocean Sciences Research Experience for Undergraduates (REU) Program.... We expect about 80 applications for 9 fellowships, but don't let that put you off. All of life is like that, and you can't get it if you don't try! If you have a decent academic record and can write an intelligible and personalized statement of interest, you stand a good chance of success.

구어적 사용역과 더 격식을 갖춘 사용역이 함께 사용된 이런 글은 지도교수가 프로페셔널할 뿐만 아니라 동시에 어떻게 독자에게 다가갈지 알고 있다는 사실을 학생들에게 보여준다.

2. 대중적 사용역(POPULAR REGISTER)

Porcupines are arboreal creatures and in the Nevada region, they live and mate in thick riparian vegetation in which it is impossible for researchers to move quietly. So, although Sweitzer has come close to catching the creatures mating, he has had to settle for stumbling upon the pairs that seem to be on the verge of reproduction — animals that provide only indirect hints about how porcupines find and pick mates. But these clues have been sufficient for Sweitzer along with fellow researcher Joel Berger of the University of Nevada, Reno, to put forward a theory that has earned them some notoriety in the select circle of experts who study this creature.

대중적 사용역은 넓은 독자층을 대상으로 하는 대중 과학잡지에 특징적으로 나타난다. 대중적 사용역을 이용한 글은 스토리를 구성하는 경우가 많으며, 이 글에서는 교미하는 고슴도치를 찾는 노력에 관한 내용이다. 이런 글에서는 독자가 그려볼 수 있는 주인공이 중요한 역할을 하며 porcupines, Sweitzer, Berger가 그런 예에 속한다. 이 글은 명료하고 이해하기 쉬우며 테크니컬 용어가 거의 없다.

3. 관습적 사용역(CONVENTIONAL REGISTER)

I tracked the movements of North American porcupines (*Erethizon dorsatum*) in the Great Basin of northwestern Nevada. I related these movements to breeding activities during the late summer and fall of 1991 and 1992. Male porcupines are polygamous and defend several females, and I hypothesized that (1) competitively dominant males would have larger home ranges than both subordinate males and adult females, and (2) the size of home ranges of adult males would vary and be positively correlated with breeding success.

관습적 사용역은 넓은 과학 독자층을 대상으로, 명료하게 쓰여진 과학저널 논문이나 박사논문, 연구제안서에 특징적으로 나타난다. 관습적 사용역은 앞의 두 사용역에 비해 더 격식을 차린 것이지만 여전히 명료하다. 이 글도 확인 가능한 주인공(I, porcupines)이 일들을 수행하는 (track, relate, defend, hypothesize) 스토리로 구성되어 있다. 이 글에는 많은 동사가 능동태로 사용되었다. 이 글은 감정적으로는 중립적이며 독자가 몇 가지 테크니컬 용어에 익숙하다고 가정하고 있다 (polygamous, dominant, subordinate, hypothesized, correlated).

4. 추상적 사용역(ABSTRACT REGISTER)

The assessment of strong directional tendencies of the North American porcupine (*Erethizon dorsatum*) in the Great Basin of northwestern Nevada was made in relation to sex-specific behavioral heterogeneity during the late summer and fall periods of 1991 and 1992. A mate-defense polygynous mating system was exhibited, and it was hypothesized that (1) comparatively larger home ranges would be defended by competitively dominant males in comparison to the home ranges of subordinate males and females and (2) male home range size variation would be positively correlated with reproductive success.

대부분의 과학자가 매일 읽고 쓰는 것이 추상적 사용역이다. 명료하지 않고 장황하며, 오만하고 지루하다. 관습적 사용역의 예문에서 사용된 주인공, I는 사라졌다. 주인공이 수행한 액션(tracked)은 "the assessment"라는 추상적 용어로 바뀌었으며 따라서 그 행위가 아무런 주인공없이 일어났다는 인상을 준다. 스토리의 요소는 사라졌다. 관습적 사용역 예문에 등장한 능동태 동사의 대부분은 수동태로 바뀌었다. 테크니컬 용어의 수가 증가했으며 긴 명사의 나열이 등장했다. 앞의 관습적 사용역 예문의 저자(이하 전자)는 "the movements of North American porcupines"를, 추상적 사용역 예문의 저자(이하 후자)는 "strong directional tendencies of the North American porcupine"을 기술하고 있다. 전자는 같은 내용을 "relates movements to breeding activities"로, 후자는 "assesses movements in relation to sex-specific behavioral heterogeneity"로 표현한다. 전자는 "the size of home ranges of adult males would vary"를 설명하고 후자는 "male home size variation"을 설명한다. 관습적 사용역으로 쓰여진 메시지는 명료하다. 왜 추상적 표현과 테크니컬 용어로 물을 흐리는가? 그렇게 하면 저자는 독자를 혼란에 또는 졸음에 빠뜨릴 위험을 감수해야 한다.

과학적 글쓰기에 부적합한 두 가지 사용역(구어적, 추상적) 중에서 추상적 사용역이 훨씬 더 흔하게 사용되며 가장 경계해야 할 대상이다. 추상적 글쓰기는 메시지를 은폐하며 독자들, 특별히 해당 주제에 익숙하지 않은 독자를 혼동시킨다.

| 어조(Tone)

어조란 자신과 자신의 주제, 독자에 대한 저자의 태도를 말한다. 어조는 오만에서 멸시, 소심함에서 자신감, 활기참에서 무미건조함, 냉소에서 긍정을 넘나들 수 있다. 올바른 어조의 선택은 독자가 여러분과 여러분의 주제에 관해 느끼는 방식을 좌우한다. 과학적 글쓰기의 어조는 가능한 중립적으로 유지해야 하지만 과학논문의 대부분이 설득을 목적으로 하기 때문에 (저자는 독자가 특정 시각이나 가설을 받아들이기 원함) 의심보다는 확신을 투사하는 어조를 선택해야 한다. 연구계획서에는 자기 확신과 열정이 필수적이기 때문에 이런 어조가 더욱 중요하다. 다음 두 글의 차이를 비교해보라. 둘 중 하나는 미국연구재단의 연구비를 성공적으로 수주한 연구계획서이다. 어조만 가지고 어떤 글이 그 계획서인지 알 수 있는가?

❶ Horned beetles could provide an opportunity to combine studies of trait development with experiments looking at sexual selection and the evolutionary significance of enlarged male weapons (horns). After almost ten years of research, the PI may now have the opportunity, if funded, to piece together disparate parts of the research program, offering opportunities to train young scientists, and possibly providing a picture of the evolution of unusual animal shapes.

❷ Horned beetles provide an unusual opportunity to combine studies of trait development with experiments exploring sexual selection and the evolutionary significance of enlarged male weapons (horns). By building on almost ten years of research directed towards this goal, the PI now has the opportunity to forge a truly integrative research program, offering unique possibilities for inspiring and training young scientists, and providing a comprehensive picture of the evolution of some of nature's most bizarre animal shapes.

첫 번째 글의 어조는 약하고 우유부단하다. 다음과 같은 동사, "could provide, may have, possibly providing"를 사용하면 확신이 없게 들린다. "if funded"와 같이 의구심을 표현하는 문구나, 연구를 "having disparate parts"로 묘사하는 것은 도움이 되지 않는다.

두 번째 글에서, 저자는 일종의 흥분과 자신감을 전달하고 있다. 단어와 어구의 미묘한 차이가 어조를 어떻게 바꾸는지 주목하라. "unusual, truly integrative, unique, comprehensive, most bizarre"와 같은 형용사 및 부사의 사용이 글을 확신에 차게 만든다. 저자는 또한 독자에게 10년간의 연구 후에 "now has the opportunity to forge a truly integrative research program"이라고 말함으로써 일종의 다급함을 전달하고 있다. 두 번째 연구는 성공한 계획서에서 발췌된 것이며 의심할 여지없이 계획서의 어조가 성공에 일조했다.

REFERENCE

1. Modified from Joos, M. The five clocks. *Int. J. Am. Linguist.* **28**, 9–2 (1962).

제3장
스토리를 말하라

스토리텔링은 인간의 독특한 특징이다. 우리는 주위 세계, 즉 과거와 현재, 미래 및 그 속에 있는 공간에 대한 지각을 발전시키기 위해 스토리를 사용한다. 다른 어떤 종류의 글도 스토리만큼 효과적으로 정보를 전달하지 못한다. 스토리텔링의 역사는 정확하게 알려져 있지 않지만 스토리텔링과 관련된 단서를 제공하는 기호학적 흔적은 적어도 칠만 년 전으로 거슬러 올라간다.

대부분의 과학자는 자신의 연구를 소통하는 것과 스토리텔링 간에 별 상관이 없다고 생각한다. 과학자는 스토리는 만들어진 것이며 과학은 사실에 기초한다고 생각한다. 하지만, 글을 쓰는 사람에게 있어서 "스토리"란 정보를 독자에게 전달하는 강력한 방법이다. 최근 연구 결과에 따르면 우리의 뇌는 주인공과 주인공의 액션으로 구성된 구조를 지닌 스토리를 인식하도록 설계되어 있다. 이런 형식으로 제시된 정보는 설득력 있고 쉽게 기억된다.[1] 과학자도 스토리의 동일한 요소, 즉 주인공과 액션을 이용해서 사실에 기초한 과학연구에 관해 글을 쓰고 마찬가지로 바람직한 결과를 얻을 수 있다. 과학연구에 관해 스토리를 쓴다고 해서 무언가를 지어내거나 감춘다는 뜻이 아니다. 오히려, 우리는 단순한 스토리의 구조에 복잡한 아이디어를 덧붙임으로써 연구를 독자뿐만 아니라 연구자 자신에게도 더 흥미진진하게 만들 수 있다.

주인공을 주어로, 액션을 동사로

어떻게 연구에 관한 스토리를 쓸 것인가? 모든 스토리에는 주인공과 액션이 있

13

다. 주인공을 문장의 주어로, 주인공의 액션을 문장의 동사로 선택함으로써 이 두 가지 요소를 충족시킬 수 있다. 여기에서 주인공이란 실제적이고 구체적인 명사, 예를 들어 sandstone, aspen trees, T cells와 같은 것이다. 주인공이 구체적일수록 주인공의 액션이 생생해지고, 더 좋은 스토리가 만들어진다. 아래에 좋은 예가 있다 (앞으로 나올 많은 예문에서도 주어에는 밑줄이 한 줄, 동사에는 밑줄이 두 줄 그어져 있다).

In the Great Lakes of Africa, large and diverse species flocks of cichlid fish have evolved rapidly. Lake Victoria, the largest of these lakes, had until recently at least 500 species of haplochromine cichlids. They were ecologically so diverse that they utilized almost all resources available to freshwater fishes in general, despite having evolved in perhaps as little as 12,400 years and from a single ancestral species. This species flock is the most notable example of vertebrate explosive evolution known today. Many of its species have vanished within two decades, which can only partly be explained by predation by the introduced Nile perch (*Lates* spp.). Stenotopic rock-dwelling cichlids, of which there are more than 200 species, are rarely eaten by Nile perch. Yet, many such species have disappeared in the past 10 years.

저자가 flocks, species, cichlids와 같이 구체적인 주어를 사용했으며 대부분 문장에서 이들 주어가 evolve, vanish, disappear와 같이 특정한 액션을 수행한다는 점에 주목하라.

과학자는 매혹적인 스토리를 가지고 있지만 이러한 스토리가 글을 통해 흥미진진하고 이해하기 쉽게 전달되는 경우는 드물다. 많은 저자가 구체적인 주인공이 아닌 추상명사를 주어로 선택한다. 추상명사는 동사나 형용사에서 유래한다. 추상명사는 만질 수 없는 아이디어, 감정, 질 등을 가리키며 이런 명사는 주인공으로서 제 역할을 못한다. 아래에는 흔히 사용되는 추상명사와 이들의 원조 동사 또는 형용사가 나열되어 있다.

동사	추상명사
understand	understanding
observe	observation
interpret	interpretation
assume	assumption
predict	prediction
manipulate	manipulation
demonstrate	demonstration
develop	development
exclude	exclusion
respond	response

형용사	추상명사
efficient	efficiency
accurate	accuracy
applicable	applicability

추상명사는 한 가지 목적에만 유용하다. 추상명사는 다른 방식으로는 여러 단어를 사용해야만 설명할 수 있는 개념을 간결하게 전달해준다. 예를 들어 evolution, facilitation, mutation과 같은 명사는 의미가 잘 확립되어 있으며 광범위한 아이디어를 하나의 단어로 농축시킨 추상명사로서 널리 받아들여지고 있다. 이런 경우와는 달리 많은 연구자들이 논문을 좀 더 복잡하게 보이게 하기 위해서 추상명사를 사용한다. 하지만 독자에게 있어서 추상명사, 특별히 주어로서 중요한 역할을 하는 추상명사는 혼란스럽다. 주어는 스토리의 주인공을 가리킨다. 문장의 주어가 구체적이 아닌 추상적 대상일 경우 독자는 주인공을 시각화할 수 없기 때문에 혼란에 빠진다.

더구나, 추상명사가 주어가 되면 문장의 주인공이 수식어나 전치사의 목적어와 같은 보조적인 역할로 전락될 수 있으며 독자는 이런 보조적인 역할을 놓치기 십상이다. 다음 예문을 살펴보자.

The behavioral <u>manifestations</u> of stress responses <u>have been shown</u> to vary greatly between individuals in rodents, pigs, birds, fish, and humans. (21 words)

이 문장의 주어는 manifestations이며, 이 추상명사는 manifest라는 동사에서 유래한다. 독자는 이런 추상적인 개념에 연결되기 어렵다. 하지만, 문장의 말미에는 피와 살이 있는 생생한 주인공이 전치사의 목적어로 등장한다: rodents, pigs, birds, fish, humans. 이러한 주인공을 주어로 전환하면 독자들이 더욱 흥미를 느끼게 될 것이다.

이 문장의 동사는 have been shown이다. 이 동사는 주인공의 액션을 그다지 잘 그려내지 못하고 있다. 하지만, 이 문장에는 몇 개의 동사가 동사가 아닌 형태로 위장해 있다. Behave (behavioral이라는 형용사로 위장), respond (responses라는 전치사의 목적어로 위장), vary (to vary라는 to 부정사 목적어로 위장). 어떤 동사가 주인공의 액션을 가장 잘 묘사하는지의 결정은 저자의 몫이지만 분명한 것은 주인공들이 수행하는 액션 중 한 가지는 behaving이라는 사실이다. 이 액션은 동사가 아니라 behavioral이라는 형용사로 표현되었으며 추상명사인 manifestations를 수식하고 있다. Behavioral을 동사인 behave로 바꾸어보자. 그러면, 갑자기 주인공들이 독자가 이해할 수 있는 무언가를 하게 된다.

Individual <u>rodents, pigs, birds, fish, and humans</u> <u>behave</u> very differently in response to stress. (14 words)

이 예문에는 구체적인 주인공이 주어로 등장한다: rodents, pigs, birds, fish, humans. 동사인 behave는 독자에게 주인공의 액션을 말해준다. 교정된 문장은 길이도 짧지만 더욱 중요한 사실은 스토리가 더욱 설득력있고 이해하기 쉽다는 점이다.

과학논문의 주인공은 현미경적 스케일에서 우주적 스케일에 이르는 다양한 형태로 등장한다.

Because of its proximity to the Milky Way, <u>NGC 205</u> presents us with an ideal opportunity to study at high linear resolution the distribution of gas in a dwarf elliptical and to investigate the effects of an interaction on the gas content and star formation history.

위 문장의 주어는 안드로메다 근처의 NGC 205라는 은하계로서 지구에서 약 300만 광년이나 떨어져 있지만 구체적인 주인공의 좋은 예를 보여준다.

다음 예문과 같이 추상명사를 주어로 사용하는 문장의 대부분은 주어를 과학자 자신으로 대치할 수 있다.

The <u>accumulation</u> of data sets from across the northern hemisphere <u>has enabled</u> us to address both the utility and cause of C and N isotope differences in ECM and SAP fungi. (31 words)

이 문장의 주어는 동사인 accumulate에서 유래한 accumulation이란 추상 명사이다. 당연히 독자는 궁금해진다. 누가 "accumulating"이란 액션을 취하고 있는가? 동사인 has enabled의 목적어인 us가 실마리를 제공한다. 이 문장에는 의미를 혼란스럽게 하는 세 개의 다른 추상명사가 사용되었다: utility, cause, differences. 문장을 명료하게 하려면 새로운 주어인 we (연구를 수행한 과학자를 가리키는)를 삽입하고 추상명사인 accumulation을 동사형인 accumulated로 바꾸라. 또한, why로 대치함으로써 두 개의 추상명사 utility, cause를 제거하라. 추상 명사 differences도 동사형 differ로 되돌릴 수 있다. 교정된 문장은 길이가 짧고 구체적이며 쉽게 이해할 수 있다.

<u>We</u> <u>analyzed</u> data sets accumulated from across the northern hemisphere to address why C and N isotopes differ in ECM and SAP fungi. (23 words)

연습문제

❶ 각 문장에서 주어에는 한 줄, 동사에는 두 줄의 밑줄을 그으라. 주어가 추상적인 가 아니면 구체적인가? 구체적인 명사를 주어로 선택하고 이들의 액션을 동사로 표 현하는 방식으로 문장을 교정하라. 그런 다음 부록2의 연습문제 해답을 참조하라.

1. Processes undertaken by diverse plants and animals are responsible for such ecological actions as nutrient cycling, carbon storage, and atmospheric regulation.

2. Declines in birth rates have been observed in many developed countries, and demographers expect that the transition to a stable population will eventually occur in many undeveloped nations as well.

3. Variations in magmatism during rifting have been attributed to variations in mantle temperature, rifting velocity or duration, active upwelling, or small-scale convection.

4. The inability of lateral variations in mantle temperature and composition, alone, to account for our observations leads us to propose that another influence was melt focusing.

5. The ability of mudrock seals to prevent CO_2 leakage is a major concern for geological storage of anthropogenic CO_2.

┃ 강력한 동사를 사용하라

동사를 추상명사로 바꾸면 문장에서 강력한 동사를 빼앗는 결과가 된다. 강력한 동사는 문장의 주인공과 그들이 하는 일 사이에 생생한 고리를 만들어 주며 따라서 독자의 흥미를 불러일으킨다. 우리는 주인공의 액션을 힘없이 묘사하는 또는 전혀 묘사하지 않는 약한 동사로 강한 동사를 대치하곤 한다. 특별히 취약한 두 개의 동사가 있다. 바로 be 동사와 have 동사다. 물론 이 두 동사는 특정 시제를 구성할 때 중요한 역할을 하며 be 동사는 아래와 같이 정의를 내릴 때 필수적이다.

The National Science Foundation and the National Institutes of Health <u>are</u> two federal agencies that fund biological research.

하지만 절대적으로 필요할 때를 제외하고는 be 동사나 have 동사를 문장의 주동사로 사용하지 말라. 이들이 등장하면 더 강력한 동사가 추상명사로 위장해 문장의 어딘가에 숨어있는 경우가 많다.

<u>Understanding seasonal habitat ranges and their distribution <u>is</u> critical for Greater Prairie Chicken conservation and management. (16 words)

이 문장의 주어는 동사구인 Understanding seasonal habitat ranges and their distribution이다. 추상명사인 Understanding은 understand, 또 다른 추상 명사인 distribution은 distribute라는 동사에서 유래한다. 전치사인 for의 목적어 는 conservation과 management이며 이 두 추상명사 역시 conserve와 manage라 는 동사에서 유래한다. 강력한 동사들이 모두 명사로 전환되었기 때문에 저자는 주 동사로 is를 사용할 수 밖에 없다. 강력한 동사(예를 들어, understand, distribute, conserve, manage)는 주인공의 액션에 관해 명료하게 소통할 수 있으며 문장에 생 동감을 부여한다. 이 문장을 교정하려면 구체적인 주인공을 주어로 소개한 뒤에 추 상명사를 강력한 동사로 되돌려 놓으라. 그러면 더 힘있고 직접적인 문장이 된다.

Before we can conserve and manage Greater Prairie Chickens, we must understand their seasonal habitats. (15 words)

교정문에서는 we must understand로 시작되는 독립절이 구체적 주어인 we (독자가 주인공으로 인식하는)와 강력한 동사인 must understand를 갖게 된다. 종속절인 Before we can conserve and manage Greter Prairie Chickens에 서는 추상명사인 conservation과 management가 강력한 동사인 can conserve and manage로 바뀌었으며 독립절과 같은 구체적 주어인 we로 시작된다.

다음 예문은 저자가 강력한 동사를 사용해 좋은 스토리텔링을 하고 있는 실례 를 보여준다.

Among the cells that bear innate immune or germline-encoded recognition receptors are macrophages, dendritic cells (DCs), mast cells, neutrophils, eosinophils, and the so-called NK cells. These cells can become activated during an inflammatory response, which is virtually always a sign of infection with a pathogenic microbe. Such cells rapidly differentiate into short-lived effector cells whose main role is to get rid of the infection; in this they mainly succeed without recourse to adaptive immunity.

첫 번째 문장은 정의이며 be 동사의 한 형태인 are를 주동사로 사용한다. 나머지 문장은 activate, differentiate, succeed와 같은 강력한 동사를 사용한다. 이런 동사들은 글을 흥미진진하게 만들고 독자를 글 속으로 끌어들인다.

❷ 각 문장에서 주동사에 밑줄을 두 줄 그으라. 약한 동사를 강한 동사를 대치함으로써 문장을 교정하라. 할 수 있는 한 추상명사를 대치하라. 그런 다음 부록2의 연습문제 해답을 참조하라.

1. Photographs from space taken by satellites are indicators of urbanization and just one of the demonstrations of the human footprint.

2. Weather variables (precipitation, temperature, and wind speed) are key factors in limiting summer habitat availability.

3. A risk management ranking system is the central mechanism for which prioritization of terrestrial invasive species is based.

4. It is clear that Prairie Chickens are closely associated with sagebrush habitat throughout the year.

5. The occurrence of freezing and thawing is an important control on cohesive bank erosion in the region.

주어와 동사를 가까이에 두라

적절한 동사의 선택만큼 적절한 동사의 위치도 중요하다. 독자는 주어를 스토리의 주인공으로 확인하는 순간 주인공의 액션을 말해주는 동사를 찾게 된다. 동사의 위치가 주어에 가까울수록 문장은 명료해진다. 아래의 잘 쓰여진 예문에서 저자는 주어 바로 뒤에 동사를 두고 있다.

Horns form during the larval period, from clusters of epidermal cells that detach from the larval cuticle and undergo a local burst of growth. In *Onthophagus taurus*, *O. nigriventris* and *Xylotrupes gideon*, the horns delay growth until very late in the larval period. As animals purge their guts in preparation for metamorphosis, these epidermal <u>cells</u> <u>begin</u> a rapid burst of proliferation and <u>form</u> evaginated discs of densely folded tissue (horn discs) that unfurl to their full length when the animal sheds its larval cuticle and molts into a pupa.

예문의 각 문장에서는 주어 바로 뒤에 동사가 등장한다: Horns form, horns delay, cells begin and form. 이렇게 하면 독자는 누가 주인공이며 주인공이 무엇을 하고 있는지 정확하게 알 수 있다.

반면에 주어 뒤의 예닐곱 단어를 훑으면서 동사를 찾아야 한다면, 주어가 무엇인지 잊게 되어 다시 앞으로 돌아오게 된다. 또한, 독자는 주어와 동사 사이의 단어를 무시하게 된다. 주어와 동사 사이에 6-7단어 이상이 끼어들어 있다면 이를 줄일 필요가 있다.

<u>Part</u> of our evidence establishing that the p65 product was derived from uncleaved FAT1 and not from the further proteolytic processing of the cleaved FAT1 heterodimer <u>was obtained</u> by the use of the furin-defective LoVo cells. (36 words)

이 문장의 주어인 Part와 동사인 was obtained 사이에는 25단어가 있다. 이 중 세 단어는 전치사구인 of our evidence로, 나머지는 주어를 수식하는 종속절인 that the p65 product was derived from uncleaved FAT1 and not from the further proteolytic processing of the cleaved FAT1 heterodimer로 이루어져 있다. 주어와 동사 사이에 이렇게 긴 훼방꾼이 있으면, 독자는 주어인 Part가 무엇을 했는지 (또는 이 경우에 무슨 일을 당했는지) 찾을 때까지 이러한 단어들을 무시하게 된다. 독자가 너무 기다리지 않도록 교정하면 다음과 같이 된다;

<u>We</u> <u>established</u> that the p65 product was not derived from the further proteolytic processing of cleaved FAT1 heterodimer. Instead, by using furin-defective LoVo cells, <u>we</u> <u>discovered</u> that p65 was derived from uncleaved FAT1. (33 words)

교정문에서는 앞의 예문이 두 개의 문장으로 나누어졌다. 각 문장에는 구체적인 주어 (we) 뒤에 강력한 동사인 established와 discovered가 뒤따른다. 교정문은 길이도 짧지만 더욱 중요한 사실은 p65의 두 가지 가능한 변종의 차이를 분명하게 드러낸다는 점이다.

연습문제

❸ 각 문장에서 주어에는 한 줄, 동사에는 두 줄의 밑줄을 그으라. 주어와 동사를 가까이 배치하라. 할 수 있는 한 추상명사를 대치하라. 그런 다음 부록2의 연습문제 해답을 참조하라.

1. Environmentally sensitive solutions to the problems associated with continued population growth and development will require an environmentally literate citizenry.
2. Partnerships between professional teachers, scientists, nonprofessional science educators, and administrators are needed to improve the content and effectiveness of science education, particularly in rural areas.
3. Our ability to predict the spatial spread of exotic species and their transformation of natural communities is still developing.
4. The amount of magmatism that accompanies the extension and rupture of the continental lithosphere varies dramatically at rifts and margins around the world.
5. The migration of melts vertically to the top of the melting region and then laterally along the base of the extended continental lithosphere would focus melts toward the eastern part of the basin.
6. Pre-treatment of tenocytes with different concentrations of wortmannin (1, 10, and 20nM) for 1 h, treated with curcumin (5μM) for 4h, and then treated with IL-1β for 1 h, inhibited the IL-1β- induced NF-κB activation.

— REFERENCE —

1. Hsu, J. The secrets of storytelling. *Scientific American Mind*, August, 46–51 (2008).

제4장

능동태를 사용하라

태(voice)란 문장의 주어가 어떤 액션을 하고 있는가 아니면 받고 있는가를 말해 준다. 문장의 주어가 어떤 액션을 하고 있으면 해당 동사는 능동태다. 주어가 어떤 액션을 받고 있으면 해당 동사는 수동태다.

| 능동태

The biologist counted the caribou. (5 words)

이 문장의 주어는 biologist이며, 동사는 counted이다. Biologist가 counting을 하고 있기 때문에 이 동사는 능동태이다.

| 수동태

The caribou were counted by the biologist. (7 words)

이 문장의 주어는 caribou이며 동사는 were counted이다. Caribou는 counting을 받는 대상이며, 따라서 이 동사는 수동태이다.

| 능동태의 장점

능동태를 사용하면 거의 모든 경우에 글이 좋아진다. 능동태 문장은 우리가 일상적으로 말하는 방식을 반영하며, 따라서 독자가 따라오기 쉽다. 능동태를 사용하면 단어 수도 적어진다. 위의 예문에서 능동태 문장이 수동태 문장에 비해 두 단어가 적다는 점에 주목하라. 능동태 문장은 직접적인 주인공-액션-목적 순으로 이루어진다. 수동태 문장에서는 이 순서가 반대가 되며 주로 -ed 또는 -en 형태로 끝나는 주동사 앞에 be 동사가 위치한다. 많은 수동태 문장이 by 구를 수반하며 이 구는 누가 액션을 취하고 있는지 설명해준다. 티끌모아 태산이다; 전체가 수동태 문장으로 이루어진 글은 능동태 문장으로 이루어진 글에 비해 길이가 30% 가량 길다. 재미있게도 저널에 투고된 많은 논문 원고에 에디터의 다음과 같은 명령이 떨어진다: "길이를 30% 줄이시오." 수동태를 능동태로 바꾸는 것이 한 가지 방법이 될 수 있다! 다음 예문을 살펴보자.

This hypothesis is supported by the observation that the timing of spring runoff is significantly different between natural and modified basins (Moore et al. 2011). (passive, 25 words)

이 예문의 주어인 hypothesis는 supporting이라는 액션을 받으며, 따라서 동사인 is supported는 수동태다. 동사를 능동태로 만들고 주어를 Moore et al. (2011)로 대치하면 be 동사를 제거할 수 있고(이 경우 is), 전치사구인 by the observations를 observing으로 줄일 수 있다. 이렇게 교정된 결과는 더 명료하고 직접적이며 단어 수가 세 개 적다.

Moore et al. (2011) support this hypothesis, observing that the timing of spring runoff is significantly different between natural and modified basins. (active, 22 words)

능동태 문장은 더 짧고 직접적일 뿐만 아니라 저자로 하여금 스토리의 주인공을 명시하도록 만든다. 수동태 문장에는 주인공이 명시되지 않는다. 주인공을 생략함으로써 여러분은 스토리텔링의 첫 번째 원칙을 위반하게 된다: 주인공을 주어로 만들라. 주인공이 없는 글은 무미건조할 뿐만 아니라 추상적이고 설득력이 떨어진다.

Dramatic improvements in policy and technology are needed to reconfigure agriculture and land use to gracefully meet global demand for both food and biofuel feedstocks. (passive, 25 words)

이 문장의 주어인 improvements는 추상명사이며 동사인 are needed는 수동태 이다. 이런 구조는 독자로 하여금 누구도 어떤 액션을 하거나 받고 있지 않다고 생각하게 만든다. 비판적인 독자라면 이렇게 물을지 모른다. "Who needs these improvements?" 더 중요하게는 "Who should reconfigure agriculture and land use so that the global demand for food and biofuel are met?" 이러한 액션의 주체가 되어야 할 주인공이 빠져 있으며 따라서 이런 충고를 따를 수도 있는 독자들이 혼란에 빠진다.

교정문에서는 저자가 미국 정부라고 가정해보자. 주어에 걸맞은 주인공과 강력한 능동태 동사를 찾으면 훨씬 직접적이고 개인적인 선언문이 만들어진다.

The Department of Agriculture must help farmers with new legislation and technology to meet global demand for biofuels without jeopardizing our food supply or environment. (active, 25 words)

이 교정문의 단어 수는 그 전과 동일하지만, The Department of Agriculture와 farmers 같이 구체적인 주인공, help라는 능동태 동사가 추가됨으로써 글이 생기를 띌 뿐만 아니라 임무가 더 급박하고 설득력있게 묘사되었다.

수동태가 추상명사와 결합하면 이해할 수 없는 문장이 탄생한다.

The variation in survivorship referred to as density-dependent mortality has also been related to negative plant-soil biota feedbacks described for a temperate (Parker and Clay 2000; Parker and Clay 2002) and tropical tree species (Hood et al. 2004). (passive, 37 words)

이 문장을 읽는 것은 마치 안개속으로 들어가는 것과 같다. 추상명사인

variation이 나약한 수동태 동사인 has been related의 주어로 등장한다. 그 다음에 등장하는 세 개의 추상명사 survivorship, mortality, feedbacks가 안개를 더욱 짙게 만든다. 주어와 동사 사이에는 여덟 개의 단어가 있다. 구체적인 명사는 모두 부수적인 역할을 담당할 뿐이다: plant, soil, biota는 feedbacks를 수식하면서 이해할 수 없는 문자열인 plant-soil biota feedbacks를 구성하고 있으며, tree는 for 전치사의 목적어인 species를 수식한다. 독자는 이렇게 질문할지 모른다. "이야기의 주인공은 누구고, 주인공이 무엇을 하고 있나요?"

교정하려면 과학자를 구체적인 주어로 사용하고 강력한 능동태 동사를 찾으라. 독자층이 흔히 사용되는 생태학 용어에 익숙하다면 density-dependent mortality를 the variation in survivorship으로 정의하지 않아도 된다. 또한, negative plant-soil biota feedbacks라는 문자열을 나누라. 하지만, 저자가 의도하는 바에 대한 추가 정보 없이는 교정문 조차도 여전히 명료하지 않다.

Parker and Clay (2000, 2002) found that density dependent mortality was related to negative feedbacks between plants and soil biota in a tropical tree species. Hood et al. (2004) found a similar relationship in a temperate tree species. (active, 37 words)

독자는 이제 누가 주인공이고 주인공이 무엇을 하고 있는지 알 수 있다. 구체적인 주어 뒤에 능동태 동사가 뒤따른다. 한 문장이 두 문장으로 나뉘었지만 교정문과 원문의 길이는 동일하다.

▌수동태의 올바른 사용법

일반적으로 능동태가 글을 더욱 명료하게 만들지만 수동태가 존재하는 몇 가지 훌륭한 이유도 있다.

첫 번째로, 수동태는 한 문단에서 일련의 문장들의 주어를 동일하게 또는 유사하게 유지시켜주는 역할을 한다(이 주제는 7장에서 다시 다루어진다). 한 문단 내의 연속되는 문장들에서 주어가 일정하게 유지되면 글을 읽고 이해하는 일이 쉬워진다.

Supernovae deposit enormous amounts of energy into their surroundings. They play a key role in the heating of their host galaxies and in the enrichment of the interstellar medium with heavy elements that form the building blocks of life. They have been well studied at radio, X-ray, infrared, and optical wavelengths, yet the actual explosion mechanism is not well understood.

저자는 이 예문에서 세 문장 모두의 주어를 Supernovae, They, They로 동일하게 유지하고 있다. 처음 두 문장의 동사는 능동태이지만 세 번째 문장에서는 주어를 일관되게 유지하기 위해서 have been studied라는 수동태 동사가 사용되었다.

두 번째로, 수동태는 강조하기 위해서 또는 앞문장의 단어와 연결하기 위해서 단어를 문장의 전략적인 부분으로 이동시킬 때 도움이 된다(이번 예문과 다른 많은 예문에서, 원칙을 예시할 때는 볼드체가 사용된다).

The fundamental constant regulating all microscopic electronic phenomena, from atomic physics to quantum electrodynamics, is the fine-structure constant α. Experimentally, the current value $α = 1/(137.03602 ± 0.00021)$ is one of the best determined numbers in physics. Theoretically, the reason why nature selects this particular numerical value has remained a mystery, and has provoked much interesting speculation. The speculations may be divided roughly into three general types.

이 예문의 첫 세 문장에는 능동태 동사가 사용되고 있다: is, is, has remained, has provoked. 세 번째 문장의 끝에는 speculation이라는 단어가 도입된다. 저자는 이렇게 새로 도입된 단어를 이어지는 문장의 새로운 주어로 매끄럽게 연결하기 위해서 may be divided라는 수동태 동사를 사용하고 있다.

마지막으로, 수동태를 사용하면 수행한 사람이 아니라 수행된 액션이 부각되는 문장을 구성할 수 있다. 과학자가 실험방법을 논할 때 이런 상황이 종종 벌어진다. 이런 경우 액션을 수행하는 사람이 너무나 분명하기 때문에 모든 문장에 이를 주어로 언급하는 것은 반복적이며 장황하다.

| 능동태

I <u>cooled</u> the samples on ice, <u>returned</u> them to Arizona State University, and <u>froze</u> them until I used them. (19 words)

| 수동태

Samples <u>were cooled</u> on ice, <u>returned</u> to Arizona State University, and <u>frozen</u> until used. (14 words)

수동태는 이런 경우 문제가 없다. 특별히 하나의 아이템이 여러 가지 다른 방식으로 다루어지는 일련의 실험에서는 단어수를 줄여주기까지 한다. 하지만, 수동태를 남용하지는 말라. 아껴서 사용하고 분명한 목적에만 사용하라. 아래 예문은 명료하고 간결하게 쓰여진 Methods 섹션에서 발췌한 글이며 능동태와 수동태 문장이 배합된 좋은 실례이다.

The <u>number</u> of animals in each chamber <u>was</u> then <u>counted</u> in one of two ways. For liberated embryos, <u>we</u> directly <u>counted</u> all embryos in each vial. For egg capsules, <u>we</u> either (1) directly <u>counted</u> embryos in all capsules and <u>summed</u> them for each vial, or (2) <u>counted</u> embryos in 20 haphazardly chosen capsules from the same mass, <u>calculated</u> the mean number of embryos per capsule, and <u>multiplied</u> the number of capsules in a given vial by this average. The latter <u>method</u> <u>was used</u> for temperature experiments because time constraints precluded immediate counts of embryos in each egg capsule.

저자는 첫 문장과 네 번째 문장에서 수동태 동사인 was counted와 was used를 사용하고 있다. 네 번째 문장에서 수동태를 사용함으로써 저자는 새로운 주어인 method를 소개하고 있으며, method는 앞 문장의 말미에 소개된 정보를 가리킨다. 두 번째, 세 번째 문장은 능동태이다. 각 문장은 For liberated embryos, For egg capsules라는 전치사구로 시작되며 이런 방식은 문장을 we로 시작하는 것의 훌륭한 대안이 된다. 첫 문장에서 수동태가 사용된 이유가 we의 남용을 막기위한 것일 수도 있다.

기억해야 할 요점은 다음과 같다. 능동태와 수동태를 선택할 때 숙고해야 한다. 수동태를 사용해야 할 좋은 이유가 있다면 그렇게 하라. 그렇지 않으면 능동태를 사용하라. 그러면, 독자들이 고마워할 것이고 여러분의 글은 더 명료하고 간결해 질 것이다.

연습문제

❹ 각 문장을 읽고 주어에는 한 줄, 동사에는 두 줄의 밑줄을 그으라. 동사가 능동태인가 수동태인가? 부록2의 연습문제 해답에서 여러분의 답이 맞는지 확인해보라.

1. Four big brown bats served as subjects in these experiments, two males and two females.
2. The animals were collected from private homes in Maryland and were housed in the University of Maryland bat vivarium.
3. Bats were maintained at 80% of their *ad lib* feeding weight and were normally fed mealworms only during experiments.
4. We exposed the bats to a reversed 12h dark: 12h light cycle, and we gave them free access to water.

연습문제

❺ 아래 문장을 수동태에서 능동태로 고치라. 원문의 단어수가 제공되고 있다. 여러분의 교정문의 단어수는 몇인가? 부록2의 연습문제 해답에서 여러분의 답이 맞는지 확인해보라.

1. For effective storage of industrial CO_2, retention times of $\sim 10^4$ yr or greater are required. (15 words)
2. It is hypothesized that groundwater pH must have been, on average, highest

shortly before the Late Ordovician to Silurian proliferation of root-forming land plants. (24 words)

3. We were compelled to rely on the SOC90 data as no further information on the occupational situation (employed vs. self-employed) or on the size of the firm was available in retrospective form. (32 words)

4. Moreover, it has been demonstrated that mineral-water reactions increase the pH of groundwater even in the presence of abundant acid-producing lichens (Schatz 1963). (24 words)

제5장
단어를 신중하게 선택하라

과학자는 길고 복잡한 단어로 표현하는 것을 좋아한다. 믿거나 말거나 이런 일이 벌어지는 이유는 11세기로 거슬러 올라간다. 당시에는 현재 잉글랜드로 알려져 있는 지방에 살던 주민들이 앵글로-색슨어 (Old English로 알려진)를 사용했다. 1066년에 잉글랜드는 프랑스 노르망디공국의 침략을 받았고 헤이스팅스 전투에서 패배했으며 이 일은 영어라는 언어에 뼛속 깊이 영향을 미쳤다. 침략 후에 노르망디인은 사회제도와 종교, 학문과 관련된 일을 좌지우지했으며 처음에는 라틴어를, 나중에는 노르망디 불어를 공식적으로 사용했다. 시간이 지나면서 라틴어와 불어 어휘가 앵글로-색슨화되면서 사회제도의 어휘목록 속에 뿌리를 내렸다. 평범한 사람들은 여전히 앵글로-색슨어를 사용했지만 식자들은 라틴어와 불어 어근을 지닌 단어로 점철된 어휘를 배웠으며 이런 어휘는 거의 예외없이 앵글로-색슨어의 동의어보다 길고 격식을 갖춘 형태였다.

르네상스 시대에는 영어 학자들이 그리스어와 라틴어 서적을 번역하면서 영어에 어휘가 없는 많은 단어를 영어화했으며 영어는 다시 한 번 확장되었다.

결과적으로 영어는 현대 유럽어 중에서 가장 유연할 뿐 아니라 형태가 다양한 언어가 되었다. 하지만, 어휘 역시 두 층으로 나뉜다. 우리가 집에서나 친구와 이야기할 때 사용되는 80% 가량의 어휘는 앵글로-색슨어, 즉 활용도가 넓고 주로 짧은 단어로 이루어진 언어에서 유래한다 (time의 뜻을 사전에서 찾아보면 무슨 말인지 알 것이다). 이러한 단어에는 the, a, this, that과 같은 관사; in, on, of, by, with같은 전치사; do, have, make, head, hand, mother, farther, sun, man, woman 등과 같이 흔히 사용되는 동사와 명사가 포함된다.

하지만, 과학 분야에서 일하고 싶다면 노르망디인이나 르네상스의 학자로부터 물려받은, 앵글로-색슨어보다 세 배나 더 양이 많고 복잡한 불어, 라틴어, 그리스어 계열의 어휘를 배워야만 한다. Anthropogenic, interpretation, attribution, demonstration과 같은 단어는 우리의 일상 경험이나 독서에 기초한 것이 아니다. 하지만, 일단 배우고 나면 더 유식해 보이기 위해서 글을 이러한 어휘로 포장하고자 하는 유혹을 누가 물리칠 수 있겠는가? 독자의 관점에서 보면 이런 행위는 아주 나쁜 글, 즉 읽기도 어렵고 이해하기도 어려운 글을 야기한다. 이러한 어휘는 분명히 쓸모가 있지만 단순한 어휘가 얼마나 명료하며 직접적인지를 잊어버리는 사람이 너무 많다.

| 긴 단어보다 짧은 단어를 사용하라

윈스턴 처칠은 이렇게 말했다. "Short words are best, and old words when short, are best of all."[1] 여기에서 처칠이 말한 "old words"는 바로 "old English words"를 말하며 처칠은 이런 단어를 글과 연설에서 사용함으로써 20세기 역사의 경로를 바꾸어 놓았다. 여러분의 생각을 독자에게 심어주고 싶다면 짧은 단어를 사용할 수 있는 곳에 라틴어나 불어에서 유래한 긴 단어를 사용하고 싶은 유혹을 견뎌야 한다. 그렇게 하면 메시지가 더욱 명료해지고 더 큰 울림이 있을 것이다. 아래에는 과학논문에 흔히 등장하는 라틴어, 불어 유래 어휘와 이들을 대치할 수 있는 간단한 대안이 제시되어 있다.

긴 단어	짧은 단어	긴 단어	짧은 단어
implement	put	transmit	send
adhere	stick	initiate	start
develop	make	alteration	change
retain	keep	investigations	work
utilize	use	prescription	plan
terminate	end	subsequent	next
ascertain	find	heterogeneous	patchy
facilitate	help	spatial	in space
endeavor	try	temporal	in time

다음 예문은 대부분의 과학논문에서 흔히 볼 수 있는 글이다.

Although investigations of medieval plague victims have identified *Yersinia pestis* as the putative etiologic agent of the pandemic, methodological limitations have prevented large-scale genomic investigations to evaluate changes in the pathogen's virulence over time. (34 words)

저자는 세 가지를 말하고 있다: *Yersinia pestis* likely caused the Black Death; not much suitable *Y. pestis* DNA is still around; and thus, large-scale genomic studies of its virulence are hard to do. 이 문장들을 더욱 복잡하게 만들기 위해서 저자는 길고 복잡한 불어, 라틴어 계열의 어휘인 investigations, identified, etiologic, methodological, limitations, evaluate을 사용하고 있다. 이 문장에 등장하는 14개의 단어가 3음절 이상이다. 더 단순하고 명료한 교정문에는 3음절 이상 단어가 5개에 지나지 않는다.

By studying medieval plague victims, we know that *Yersinia pestis* likely caused the Black Death; however, we don't know how the pathogen's virulence changed over time, because large-scale genomic studies are hard to do. (34 words)

이 교정문에서 나는 길고 복잡한 단어의 상당수를 짧은 단어인 know, likely, caused, how, hard, do로 대치했다. 여러분은 어쩌면 다른 개선점을 이미 발견했는지 모르겠다. 나는 추상적인 주어인 limitations를 구체적인 명사인 we로 대치했다.

물리학의 전설적인 논문에서 발췌한 아래 예문을 보면 저자는 짧고 친숙한 단어를 사용해서 복잡한 주제를 설명한다: the physics of organisms moving in viscous liquids. 글이 얼마나 명료한지 보라.

There is a very funny thing about motion at low Reynolds number, which is the following. One special kind of swimming motion is what I call a reciprocal motion. That is to say, I change my body into a certain shape and then I go back to the original shape by going through the sequence in reverse. At low Reynolds number, everything reverses just fine. Time, in fact, makes no difference—only configuration. If I change quickly or slowly, the pattern of motion is exactly the same.

이 예문에 사용된 87개 단어 중에서 65%가 하나의 음절만을 갖는다: shape, thing, time과 같은 명사; be, change, say, go, make와 같은 동사; of, at, by, in 과 같은 전치사; which, what, that과 같은 대명사. 이런 단어의 대부분은 Old English에서 유래한 것이다. 우리는 이런 단어를 매일 서로 이야기할 때 사용한다. 특별한 이유가 없는 한 글을 쓸 때도 그렇게 해야한다.

연습문제

ⓖ 연습문제에서 밑줄이 그어진 단어 각각의 음절은 몇 개인가? 이 단어들이 라틴어, 불어 또는 오래된 영어(old English)에서 기원한 것인지 구별할 수 있는가? 각 단어의 어원을 찾은 다음 의미를 훼손하지 않는 범위 내에서 old English 단어를 가능한 많이 사용해 문장을 다시 쓰라. 대치한 더 짧은 단어의 음절수와 어근을 나열하라. 부록2의 연습문제 해답에서 여러분의 답이 맞는지 확인해보라.

1. For example, <u>expansion</u> of the extent of the winter range by <u>continued</u> <u>pioneering</u> of segments of the northern Yellowstone elk herd northward from the park <u>boundary</u> and <u>extensive</u> use of these more northerly areas by greater numbers of elk have been <u>coincident</u> with <u>acquisition</u> and <u>conversion</u> of rangelands from livestock <u>production</u> to elk winter range.
2. We conclude that snag <u>retention</u> at <u>multiple</u> <u>spatial</u> and <u>temporal</u> scales in recent burns, which will be salvage-logged, is a <u>prescription</u> that must be <u>implemented</u> to meet the <u>principles</u> of <u>sustainable</u> forest <u>management</u> and the <u>maintenance</u> of biodiversity in the boreal forest.

| 용어를 동일하게 유지하라

많은 저자들이 주인공에 대해 동일한 용어를 사용하면 글이 지루하고 반복적이 된다고 믿는다. 그래서, 대신에 다른 용어들을 혼용하곤 한다. 이렇게 하면 독자는 저자가 서로 다른 대상을 의미한다고 생각하기 쉽다. 독자에게 있어서 일관성있는 용어의 사용은 지루한 것과는 전혀 다르다. 용어의 일관성은 새롭고 복잡한 정보를 항해하는 일에 필수적이다.

In relatively unproductive ecosystems like deserts, **grazers** and **predators** are so rare as to be negligible, and competition for resources structures **plant communities**. In more productive systems like grasslands, a large effective **herbivore community** can be supported and grazing determines **plant biomass**. (42 words)

저자는 이 글에서 deserts와 grasslands라는 두 개의 생태계를 비교하면서 각 생태계의 식생을 제한하는 요소를 설명한다. 이런 비교는 독자가 이해하기 어렵다. 왜냐하면 두 개 이상의 상황을 기억하면서 머릿속으로 서로를 비교해야 하기 때문이다. 같은 대상에 다른 용어가 사용되는 것처럼 비교를 흐리게 하는 요소가 있으면 더욱 그렇다. 이 글에서는 주인공과 관련된 용어가 다르다: 첫 문장의 plant communities와 두 번째 문장의 plant biomass. 저자는 같은 대상을 지칭하고 있는가? Herbivores 역시 중요한 주인공이지만 두 가지 형태로 나타난다: grazers, herbivore community. Predators 역시 중요하지만 한 번 언급된 후 사라진다. 이 주인공은 스토리에 필수적인가? 대부분의 독자는 이런 글을 그럭저럭 이해하고 넘어가겠지만 저자는 독자에게 별 도움을 주지 못했다. 독자의 집중력은 서로 다른 용어를 헤쳐나가기 위해 계속해서 분산된다. 교정을 위해서는 일관적인 용어로 주인공을 언급하라.

In relatively unproductive ecosystems like deserts, **plant biomass** is limited by a lack of resources. In more productive systems like grasslands, **plant biomass** is limited by herbivores. (27 words)

이제 독자는 두 생태계를 쉽게 비교할 수 있다. 두 문장의 주인공은 동일하다: plant biomass. 이 주인공은 deserts에서는 resource가 부족하기 때문에, grasslands 에서는 herbivores 때문에 제한된다. 만약 predators도 중요하다면 이 주인공은 별도의 문장을 이용해 설명할 수 있다.

연습문제

❼ 연습문제의 문장에서 같은 대상을 가리키는 서로 다른 용어를 찾고 밑줄 그으라. 서로 다른 용어를 동일한 뜻을 가진 단어들로 대치하라. 가능한 짧고 단순한 단어를 활용하라. 부록2의 연습문제 해답에서 여러분의 답이 맞는지 확인해보라.

1. One way to assess the perceived risk of feeding in different locations is to measure the proportion of the available food a forager removes before switching to an alternative patch. All else being equal, foragers should be willing to forage longer and remove more food from a safe area than a risky one.

2. Stress coping styles have been characterized as a proactive/reactive dichotomy in laboratory and domesticated animals. In this study, we examined the prevalence of proactive/reactive stress coping styles in wild-caught short-tailed mice (*Scotinomys teguina*). We compared stress responses to spontaneous singing, a social and reproductive behavior that characterizes this species.

3. Antimicrobial resistance genes allow a microorganism to expand its ecological niche, allowing its proliferation in the presence of certain noxious compounds. From this standpoint, it is not surprising that antibiotic resistance genes are associated with highly mobile genetic elements, because the benefit to a microorganism derived from antibiotic resistance is transient, owing to the temporal and spatial heterogeneity of antibiotic-bearing environments.

4. Studies of long-term outcomes in offspring exposed to maternal undernutrition and stress caused by the Dutch Hunger Winter of 1944 to 1945 revealed an increased prevalence of metabolic disease, such as glucose intolerance, obesity, and cardiovascular disease, as well as emotional and psychiatric disorders. Animal models have been developed to assess the long-term consequences

of a variety of maternal challenges including under- and overnutrition, hyperglycemia, chronic stress, and inflammation. Exposures to a wide range of insults during gestation are associated with convergent effects on fetal growth, neurodevelopment, and metabolism.

| 명사열을 쪼개라

과학논문 저자에게는 또 다른 나쁜 습관이 있다: 명사들을 길고 거추장스럽게, 때로는 수식어까지 덧붙여서 묶어놓는 것. 명사열은 그 중의 어떤 단어가 중요한지 알 수 없기 때문에 독자가 이해하기 어렵다. 이 문제에 있어서는 길이만큼이나 친숙도가 중요하다. 짧고 친숙한 명사열은 유용할 때가 있다. 이런 명사열은 population dynamics와 같이 복잡한 개념을 소수의 단어로 표현하게 해준다. 독자가 이런 명사열에 익숙하다면, 그리고 이런 명사열의 사용으로 단어수를 줄일 수 있다면 사용하라. 하지만 평소 접하기 어려운 긴 명사열의 사용은 피하라.

As the **labor market time commitment** of mothers has increased in western societies in the recent decades, <u>questions</u> about the provisions of care for children, especially in relation to maintaining and generating time for care, <u>have attracted</u> **significant international social and policy attention.** (43 words)

이 문장은 네 단어로 구성된 명사열로 시작된다. labor market time commitment는 As로 시작되는 종속절의 주어이다. 독자는 자연스럽게 이런 질문을 던지게 된다. 네 단어 중 어떤 명사가 mothers를 가장 잘 설명하는가?; mothers' labor, mothers' time, mothers' commitment? 다른 질문들도 많다; 종속절의 주어인 questions는 추상적이며 동사인 have attracted와 열일곱 단어나 떨어져 있다. 목적어인 attention은 네 개의 수식어 때문에 옴짝달싹 못한다: significant, international, social, policy. 교정을 위해서는 명사열을 쪼개서 워킹맘의 삶의 한 단면이며 글의 논의에 가장 적절한 "time"을 강조하라. 추상적인 주어를 구체적인 명사로 대치한 뒤 동사를 가까이에 두라. 그런 다음 attention의 수식어를 재배치해서 글을 더 명료하게 만들라.

As mothers in western societies commit more time to work, <u>they spend</u> less time with their children. This <u>phenomenon has attracted</u> widespread attention from social scientists and policy makers. (29 words)

이 교정문에서 나는 추상명사인 commitment를 동사인 commit로, 명사열인 labor market time을 to의 힘을 빌어 as mothers … commit more time to work로 바꾸었다. 이제 구체적인 주어인 they 바로 뒤에 동사인 spend가 등장하며 attention의 수식어는 from의 힘을 빌어 나누었다. 교정문은 두 개의 문장이 되었지만 원문보다 단어수가 14개 줄었다.

연습문제

❸ 아래의 문장에서 명사열에 밑줄을 그은 뒤 명사열을 쪼개고 긴 단어를 짧은 단어로 대치함으로써 문장을 교정하라. 부록2의 연습문제 해답에서 여러분의 답이 맞는지 확인해보라.

1. Developing regular exercise programs and diet regimes contributes to disease risk prevention and optimal health promotion.
2. Research focused on care time deficits and time squeezes for families has identified the persistence of gendered care time burdens and the sense of time pressure many dual-earner families experience around care.
3. There will be major conservation implications if mercury ingestion in ospreys causes negative population level effects either through direct mortality or negative fecundity.

| 테크니컬 용어는 두 번 생각하라

이 책에서 사용되는 테크니컬 용어의 의미는 특정 전문분야나 연구분야 그룹 내에서만 통용되는 용어를 말한다. 테크니컬 용어는 과학의 특징 중 하나이며 과학분야가 점점 세분화되면서 이를 설명하기 위해 새로운 용어들이 만들어진다. 이러한 용어는 해당 분야 안에서는 복잡한 아이디어를 짧고 효율적으로 표현하게 해주지만 분야 밖의 사람은 이해하기 어렵다. 내가 만난 한 면역학자는 면역학의 다른 세부 분야의 동료들이 쓴 논문을 면역학인 본인도 이해하기 어렵다고 말했다!

부동산 업자들은 부동산을 살 때 가장 중요한 요소로 "location, location, location"을 꼽는다. 마찬가지로 논문의 저자는 글을 쓸 때 가장 중요한 요소로 "audience, audience, audience"를 꼽아야 한다. 테크니컬 용어는 모든 독자가 해당 용어를 이해한다는 확신이 있을 때만 사용하라. DNA나 3D와 같은 테크니컬 용어는 거의 모든 사람이 이해하고 있으며 설명이 필요없다. 독자들이 얼마나 알고 있는지 자신이 없다면 보수적으로 행동하라. 테크니컬 용어를 정의하거나 사용하지 말라.

Aneuploidy and translocations lead to progressive alterations in chromosome structure and epigenetic modifications characteristic of tumorigenesis. (16 words)

이 예문은 유전학 분야의 테크니컬 용어를 담고 있다: Aneuploidy, translocations, epigenetic modifications, tumorigenesis. 고급 유전학에 익숙한 독자만이 이런 용어를 이해할 수 있다. 유전학 분야 지식이 제한된 독자에게 이 문장은 해독이 불가능하다. 더 넓은 독자층을 위해 테크니컬 용어를 최소화하자면 다음과 같다.

Relative to the cell lines from which they arose, cells prone to become tumors characteristically show abnormal chromosome numbers, chromosomal rearrangements, and aberrant patterns of gene expression arising from defects in gene regulation. (33 words)

이 교정문은 테크니컬 용어를 이해하는 사람에게 테크니컬 용어가 유용한 이유를 보여준다. 교정문은 원문보다 단어가 두 배 많으며, chromosomal rearrangement, gene expression, gene regulation과 같이 설명하고자 하면 서너 문장이 추가로 소요되는 용어를 여전히 포함하고 있다. 테크니컬 용어를 이용하면 분명히 단어수를 줄일 수 있다. 하지만 이런 용어를 이해하지 못할 수 있는 독자를 대상으로 글을 쓴다면 테크니컬 용어를 정의하거나 사용하지 말라. 다음 예문을 살펴보자.

Several entities have petitioned for Prairie Chicken listing consideration under the ESA, and the USFWS responded to this with a positive 90-day finding in 2005. (25 words)

ESA, USFWS, a positive 90-day finding과 같은 용어는 Endangered Species Act 를 이해하는 사람에게는 친숙할 것이다. 그렇지 않은 독자에게는 이 문장의 의미 가 분명하지 않다. 교정문에서는 독자에게 테크니컬 용어의 의미를 설명하거나 제거하자.

Several groups have petitioned the United States Fish and Wildlife Service (USFWS) to list Prairie Chickens under the Endangered Species Act (ESA). The USFWS has responded within the mandated period of 90 days that listing is warranted. (37 words)

교정문에서는 USFWS와 ESA라는 약어가 정의되었고 법률용어인 a positive 90-day finding이 설명되었다. 이렇게 한 뒤에는 독자를 혼동시키지 않고 테크니 컬 용어를 사용할 수 있다.

다음 예문은 넓은 과학독자층을 지닌 저널에 실린 잘 쓰여진 서론의 한 문단이 다. 저자는 용어를 잘 정의함으로써 다른 분야의 독자가 개념을 이해할 수 있도록 했다.

Many biological systems have evolved to work with a very high energetic efficiency. . . . At first glance, the beating of cilia and flagella does not fall into the category of processes with such a high efficiency. Cilia are hair-like protrusions that beat in an asymmetric fashion to pump the fluid in the direction of their effective stroke. They propel certain protozoa, such as *Paramecium*, and also fulfill a number of functions in mammals including mucous clearance from airways, left-right asymmetry determination, and transport of an egg cell in fallopian tubes.

Cilia를 정의하고 그 기능을 설명함으로써 저자는 독자가 논문의 나머지를 이해할 수 있도록 준비시킨다. 논문의 나머지 부분은 cilia 운동의 에너지 효율을 측정하는 방법과 최적의 운동패턴을 계산하는 방법을 소개한다.

연습문제

😊 다음에는 면역학 분야의 복잡한 예문이 제시되어 있다. 저자가 면역학 분야의 넓은 독자층이 논문을 이해할 수 있도록 노력했는가? 그렇다면 성공했는가? 성공했다면, 또는 실패했다면 이유는? 부록2의 연습문제 해답에서 여러분의 답이 맞는지 확인해보라.

I. One of the well-researched immunoregulatory functions of probiotics is the induction of cytokine production. In particular, the induction of IL-10 and IL-12 production by probiotics has been studied intensively, because the balance of IL-10/IL-12 secreted by macrophages and dendritic cells in response to microbes is crucial for determination of the direction of the immune response. IL-10 is an anti-inflammatory cytokine and is expected to improve chronic inflammation, such as that of inflammatory bowel disease and autoimmune disease. IL-10 downregulates phagocytic and T cell functions, including the production of proinflammatory cytokines, such as IL-12, TNF-α, and IFN-γ, that control inflammatory responses. IL-10 promotes the development of regulatory T cells for the control of excessive immune responses. In contrast, IL-12 is an important mediator of cell-mediated immunity and is expected to augment the natural immune defense against infections and cancers. IL-12 stimulates T cells to secrete IFN-γ, promotes Th1 cell development, and, directly or indirectly, augments the cytotoxic activity of NK cells and macrophages. IL-12 also suppresses redundant Th2 cell responses for the control of allergy.

═ REFERENCE ═══════════════════════

1. Churchill, W. An elder statesman as man of letters. *New York Times Magazine*, Nov. 13, 78–79 (1949).

제6장
불필요한 단어는 생략하라

과학논문은 때로 장황하다. 우리는 내용도 복잡한데다 글까지 장황한 논문을 읽어야 하는 엄청난 임무를 감내해왔다. 저자로서 우리의 목표는 가지고 있는 생각을 잉여분의 단어 없이 표현하는 것이며 이는 독자가 쉽게 추론할 수 있는 것을 생략함으로써 가능하다.

쉬운 영어로 글을 쓰면 글이 간결해지는 장점이 있다. 우리가 교정한 글의 대부분이 원문보다 짧다는 점을 기억하라. 지금까지 우리가 논의한 원칙을 적용할 경우 장황한 글이 어떻게 간결해질 수 있는지 아래 예문을 살펴보자.

Inhalation of vapor phase particulate matter chemical contaminants from biomass combustion in domestic settings is a significant contributor to local disease burden. (22 words)

이 문장에는 여러 가지 문제가 있다. 주어인 Inhalation은 추상명사이며 inhale이라는 동사에서 유래한다. 그 뒤에는 세 개의 전치사구가 등장한다: of vapor phase particulate matter chemical contaminants (which contains a string of six nouns), from biomass combustion, in domestic settings. 주어와 동사 사이에는 열세 개의 단어가 존재한다. 동사인 is는 약하다. 이 문장에 생동감을 줄 수 있는 강력한 동사는 명사형으로 바뀌었다: inhale은 inhalation, combust는 combustion, contribute는 contributor로.

또한 저자는 아주 단순한 개념을 설명하기 위해 저자가 생각할 수 있는 가장 복잡한 단어를 사용하고 있다: vapor phase particulate matter chemical contaminants

의 의미는 smoke이며, biomass combustion은 burning, is a significant contributor 는 causes, disease burden은 health problems를 의미한다. 쉬운 영어의 원칙을 적용 함으로써 우리는 다음과 같이 명료하고 간결한 문장을 얻게된다.

Domestic wood <u>smoke</u> <u>causes</u> local health problems. (7 words)

Smoke는 구체적인 명사이며 causes는 강력한 동사다. 명사열은 쪼개졌고 독자 가 이해할 수 있는 단어로 대치되었다. 주어와 동사가 손에 손을 잡고 있다. 교정 문은 일곱 개 단어로 구성되어 있으며, 원문의 22단어에 비해 3분의 1 길이다!

| 중복성

논문을 부풀리는 불필요한 어휘의 대부분은 중복되는 단어, 즉 제거하더라도 메시지 전달에 아무런 해가 없는 단어들이다. 중복성은 다양한 형태로 나타나며 가장 흔한 형태 중 몇 가지를 다음에 소개하고자 한다.

1. 반복

한 번에 명료하게 기술하는 대신 살짝 다른 어휘를 이용해서 같은 내용을 반복 하는 경우가 있다. 이러면 단어가 낭비되고 요점이 흐려진다.

Despite the widely recognized importance of instream wood and organic debris dams in forested stream ecosystems, analytical approaches to quantify the spatial extent and pattern of instream wood distribution are rare and the usefulness of available metrics has been seldom evaluated. Wood influences stream geomorphology, biotic habitat, and biogeochemical cycling, therefore quantifying the spatial distribution of instream wood is important for understanding the corresponding distribution of key stream functions. (69 words)

위 단락의 요점 리스트는 다음과 같다.

1. Wood in streams is important.
2. Ways to measure wood in streams are few and seldom evaluated.

3. Because it affects stream functions, wood in streams is important.
4. Because it affects stream functions, measuring wood in streams is important.

이렇게 정리해 놓으면 무엇이 반복되는지 쉽게 알 수 있다. 요점 중 하나인 wood in streams is important가 반복되고 있으며 다른 요점인 measuring wood in streams is important는 말하지 않아도 자명하다. 약간의 재조직 및 단순화를 통해 반복을 제거할 수 있으며 그 결과로 명료하고 간결한 글을 얻을 수 있다.

Pieces of wood and the dams they produce influence stream geomorphology, biotic habitat, and biogeochemical cycling. Despite this, there are few methods for measuring wood in streams, and these are seldom evaluated. (32 words)

2. 과도한 세부사항
독자에게 과도한 세부사항을 전달하고자 할 때도 있다.

Nature is ripe with examples of the exquisite mechanisms organisms utilize to salvage survivorship in the face of unfortunate circumstances, and regeneration is one such process. Regeneration is a way that stick insects cope with shedding a limb to survive either fouled molt or a predation attempt, but like other organisms, this process often comes with associated costs. (58 words)

이 초록의 첫 문장에서 저자는 nature나 exquisite mechanisms, unfortunate circumstances에 관해 언급하지 않고도 regeneration을 더 간결하게 설명할 수 있었다. 저자가 뒤에서 자세히 설명하고자 하지 않는다면 두 번째 문장에서 다른 organisms과 비교하는 일 역시 불필요하다. 교정문은 과도한 세부사항 없이 요점만을 기술하고 있다.

Many organisms regrow lost limbs through a process called regeneration. In stick insects, regeneration allows individuals to survive a predation attempt or a fouled molt, but at a cost. (29 words)

분명한 사실은 저자가 제공해야 하는 세부사항의 수준은 독자의 지식 수준과 글의 목적에 따라 달라진다는 점이다. 예를 들어, 같은 주제라도 학생이 숙제로 제출할 보고서에서는 교수가 학술지에 쓰는 것보다 훨씬 많은 세부사항이 담겨야 한다. 독자가 다르기 때문이다: 학생은 학생의 지식을 평가할 교수를 위해 쓰는 것이고, 교수는 지식이 풍부한 독자를 대상으로 한다.

3. 하나의 어구를 하나의 단어로 대치하라

논문 저자들은 훨씬 간결하게 표현될 수 있는 내용에 습관적으로 장황한 어구를 사용한다. 이런 어구는 너무 널리 사용되기 때문에 어떤 저널의 에디터들은 이런 어구를 목록으로 만들기까지 했다. 저명한 저널의 에디터는 장황한 어구 목록과 간결한 대안을 아래 목록과 같이 제공했다.[1]

장황한 어구	간결한 대안
in this study we assessed	we assessed
conduct an investigation of	investigate
were responsible for	caused
played the role of	were
in order to	to
for the following reasons	because
during the course of; during the process of	during
a majority; most of the	most
undertake an examination of	study
various lines of evidence	evidence
the analysis presented in this paper	our analysis
in the absence of	without
located in; located at	in; at

in the vicinity of; in close proximity to	near
in no case; on no occasion	never
at the present time; at this point in time	now
an example of this is the fact that	for example

장황한 어구는 쉽게 제거할 수 있다. 문제는 이들을 인식할 수 있는지 여부다.

4. "THE"

정관사 "the"는 의미의 훼손없이 생략 가능한 경우가 많다. 앞 장의 예문에도 그런 예가 있다.

Certainly, **the** merit of your scientific writing rests as much on **the** content as on **the** style. Equally important are **the** questions, **the** hypotheses, **the** experimental designs, and **the** interpretations you describe. (32 words)

the를 상당수 제거하면 더 짧고 힘있는 문장이 된다.

Certainly, the merit of your scientific writing rests as much on content as on style. Equally important are the questions, hypotheses, experimental designs, and interpretations you describe. (27 words)

| 연결어구의 사용

우리는 좋은 효과를 내기 위해 거의 모든 글에서 연결어구를 사용한다: 의견을 추가하기 위해서는 I believe, to summarize, in conclusion과 같은 어구를, 글을 구조화하기 위해서는 first, second, more importantly와 같은 어구를, 독자를 안내하기 위해서는 note that, in order to understand, consider now와 같은 연결어구를 사용한다.

연결어구는 도로표지판과 같다. 독자는 표지판을 보면서 문장 및 단락 사이를 매끄럽게 연결할 수 있다. 잘만 사용하면 글이 술술 읽힌다. 다음 예문은 연결어구가 바람직한 목적으로 사용된 실례를 보여준다.

Dorsal, which is activated by the Toll pathway during dorso-ventral axis formation, does not appear to play a role in the systemic immune response in adult flies. **Instead**, another NF-κB family member — Dif (drosophila immunity factor) — is required for the induction of Drosomycin by Toll. **Additionally**, Spatzle is required for the activation of Toll by fungal pathogens; **however**, the serine protease cascade that generates active Spatzle during development is not involved in the immune response. **Therefore**, a different protease cascade must regulate its processing.

이 예문에서 저자는 instead, additionally, however, therefore와 같은 연결어구를 사용함으로써 복잡한 발달 과정 속에서 독자를 안내해준다.

연결어구는 거의 모든 글에서 어느 정도 필요하지만, 과도하면 아이디어 자체가 묻힐 수 있다. 과도함과 적절함의 차이를 알기란 쉽지 않으며 특정 분야에 새로 진입한 저자의 경우 더욱 그렇다.

In this essay I will be talking about how forest fragmentation causes declines in neotropical migrants. **The particular articles that I read for this essay really gave me a good idea of the background of this issue. It is well known that** neotropical migrants are declining because of deforestation in their wintering habitat, **but what was new to me was learning that** forest fragmentation in eastern North America was also detrimental. (71 words)

저자는 논문의 서론에서 많은 연결어구를 이용해 아이디어를 뒤덮고 있다: In this essay I will be talking about how, The particular articles I read for this essay really gave me a good idea of the background of this issue, It is well known that, but what was new to me was learning that. 이들 중 일부는 정제되어야 하고 일부는 남을 수도 있다. 예를 들어, 지도교수는 저자가 수집한 정보가 저자의 시각을 어떻게

바꾸었는지 궁금해할 수도 있다. 연결어구를 어느 정도 남겨놓으면 대화체 어조를 만드는 효과도 있다.

It is well known that neotropical migrants are declining because of deforestation in their wintering habitat, **but what was new to me was learning that** forest fragmentation in eastern North America was also detrimental. (34 words)

나는 첫 두 문장에서 불필요한 연결어구와 반복되는 정보를 제거했다 (forest fragmentation이 neotropical migrants 감소를 초래한다는 사실을 두 번 언급할 필요는 없다). 하지만, 대화체 어조를 만들고 학생이 배운 바를 강조하기 위해서 세 번째 문장의 연결어구는 남겨두었다.

다음과 같이 불필요한 연결어구는 독자를 지치게 한다.

In the previous section of this paper, I concluded that the problem of rising sea levels was important. **In this next** section, I would like to describe the additional problem of ocean acidification. (33 words)

위 예문은 아래와 같이 바꿀 수 있다:

The next problem is ocean acidification. (6 words)

어떤 연결어구는 글에 불특정한 관찰자를 남겨둔다. 교정문에서는 관찰결과만을 언급하도록 하라.

High birth rates **have been observed** to occur in parts of the Midwest that **have been determined** to have especially high rates of unemployment. (24 words)

위의 예문은 아래와 같이 바꿀 수 있다:

High birth rates occur in parts of the Midwest that have especially high rates of unemployment. (16 words)

연결어구의 또 다른 원천은 모호한 표현과 강조 표현이다. 이러한 표현은 신중함 또는 자신감을 전달할 때 사용된다. 이러한 표현이 과도하면 글이 장황해지고 과학자이자 저자로서 안 좋은 인상을 독자에게 심어준다.

모호한 표현에는 usually, often, sometimes, perhaps, may, might, can, could, seem, suggest와 같은 단어가 포함된다. 모호한 표현이 실제 불확실성을 전달할 때도 있지만, 불필요하게 사용하면 스스로 확신이 없는 것처럼 들린다.

We found that juveniles **were more likely to move** towards the speaker, approaching closer and more quickly, during the simulated song interactions than during solo song or control playback trials. These results **indicate** that juveniles are especially interested in eavesdropping on song contests and **suggest** that these types of social interactions **may be** particularly powerful tutoring events.

이 예문에 사용된 were more likely to move, indicate, suggest, may be와 같은 동사는 이 연구의 결과가 확정적이지 않다는 인상을 심어준다. 하지만, 이 연구의 결과는 가설을 강력하게 뒷받침하고 있으며 따라서 소심하게 표현할 이유가 없다.

We found that juveniles **were particularly attracted** to countersinging interactions and approached playbacks of these song interactions **significantly more** than simulated solo singing or the control playback trials. This result **is consistent** with the social eavesdropping hypothesis that juveniles **may learn** to sing via eavesdropping on the singing interactions of adults.

위의 교정문에 사용된 동사와 수식어는 더 강력하고 단정적이다: were particularly attracted, significantly more, is consistent. 이 교정문은 결과가 확정적이라는 확신을 독자에게 심어준다.

모호한 표현을 신중하게 사용해야 하는 또 한 가지 이유는 과도하게 한정할 수 있기 때문이다. 위에 제시된 원문의 마지막 문장을 다시 살펴보자.

These results **indicate** that juveniles are especially interested in eavesdropping on song contests and **suggest** that these types of social interactions **may be** particularly powerful tutoring events.

이 문장에는 세 개의 한정어가 존재한다: indicate, suggest, may be. 하나의 한정어 (suggest) 만으로도 같은 수준의 불확실성을 전달할 수 있기 때문에 그렇게 많이 포함시킬 필요가 없다.

These results **suggest** that juveniles are especially interested in eavesdropping on song contests and that these types of social interactions are particularly powerful tutoring events.

강조 표현은 모호한 표현의 반대다. 강조 표현에는 clearly, very, obviously, indeed, undoubtedly, certainly, major, primary, essential과 같은 단어가 포함된다. 과학논문에 자주 등장하지는 않지만 등장할 때는 신선하다. 강조 표현은 중요한 정보를 부각시키기 때문에 독자가 친숙하지 않은 주제를 이해하는 데 도움이 된다. 강조 표현은 2장에서 언급된 예문처럼 경쟁해야 하는 연구계획서를 쓸 때 더 중요하다.

Horned beetles provide an **unusual** opportunity to combine studies of trait development with experiments exploring sexual selection and the evolutionary significance of enlarged male weapons (horns). By building on almost ten years of research directed towards this goal, the PI now has the opportunity to forge a **truly integrative** research program, offering **unique** possibilities for inspiring and training young scientists, and providing a **comprehensive** picture of the evolution of some of nature's **most bizarre** animal shapes.

이 예문에서는 unusual, truly integrative, unique, comprehensive, most bizarre와 같은 강조 표현이 평가자에게 이 프로젝트가 연구비를 지원할 만한 가치가 있다는 확신을 심어주는 데 일조하고 있다.

| 긍정적 표현과 부정적 표현

긍정적 표현은 부정적 표현에 비해 단어수가 적은 경우가 많다. 긍정적 문장에서는 주어가 다른 무언가에 무언가를 하지만, 부정적 문장에서는 주어가 다른 무언가에 무언가를 하지 않는다. 부정적인 문장은 무엇이 아니라는 것을 말함으로써 일어나고 있는 일을 나타내려고 하기 때문에 불투명하다. 긍정적인 문장은 요점을 더 직접적으로 나타낸다. 물론, 여러분이 어떤 논점을 반대하거나 부정하는 문장에서는 부정적 표현만이 가능할 것이다. 하지만, 부정적 표현의 상당수를 긍정적 표현으로 재구성함으로써 단어를 절약할 수 있다. 아래 목록에 몇 가지 예가 있다.

부정적 표현	긍정적 표현
did not accept	rejected
did not consider	ignored
does not have	lacks
did not allow	prevented
not the same	different
not possible	impossible
not many	few

다음 예문에서는 저자가 부정적 표현을 이용해 논점을 제기하고 있다.

The canopy cover of Norway maples **does not allow** sufficient light to penetrate the understory and native tree seedlings **cannot germinate**. (21 words)

두 개의 부정적 표현(does not allow, cannot germinate)을 상응하는 긍정적 표현으로 바꾸면 글이 더 직접적이 되고 단어수를 하나 절약할 수 있다.

The canopy cover of Norway maples **blocks** sufficient light from penetrating the understory and **prevents** native tree seedlings from germinating. (20 words)

단어는 너무나 쉽게 불어나기 때문에 간결한 과학논문은 희귀할 뿐 아니라 실제로 주목할 만한 가치가 있다. 한 가지 유명한 예로는 J. D. Watson과 F. H. C. Crick이 DNA의 구조에 대해 쓴 한 페이지짜리 논문이 있으며 아래 예문은 거기에서 발췌되었다.[2]

We wish to put forward a radically different structure for the salt of deoxyribose nucleic acid. This structure has two helical chains each coiled round the same axis (see diagram). We have made the usual chemical assumptions, namely, that each chain consists of phosphate diester groups joining β-D-deoxyribofuranose residues with 3′, 5′ linkages. The two chains (but not their bases) are related by a dyad perpendicular to the fibre axis. Both chains follow right-handed helices, but owing to the dyad the sequences of the atoms in the two chains run in opposite directions.

연습문제

⑩ 연습문제의 예문에서 문장과 단락이 장황한 이유를 설명하라. 불필요한 단어를 가능한 많이 제거함으로써 교정하라. 원문의 단어수가 제시되어 있다. 여러분의 교정문의 단어수는 몇인가? 부록2의 연습문제 해답에서 여러분의 답이 맞는지 확인해보라.

1. While a growing body of research indicates that large herbivores as a group can exert strong indirect effects on co-occurring species, there are comparatively few

examples of strong community-wide impacts from individual large herbivore species. (37 words)

2. Small mammal species diversity increased in exclosures relative to controls, while survivorship showed no significant trends. (16 words)

3. In this essay, I will be looking at how higher summer temperatures cause quicker soil and plant evaporation. We all know that climate change has caused elevated temperatures in the Northwest throughout the spring and summer months. We also know that these record-breaking temperatures have the effect of quickly and easily desiccating soil and drying out plant foliage so that it is more flammable. Understandably then, when lightning strikes this very combustible environment, a spark can very quickly turn into a widespread blaze. (83 words)

4. Zimbabwean undocumented migrants are shown to be marginalized and vulnerable with limited transnational citizenship. (14 words)

5. When the lithosphere extends and rifts along continental margins, magma is produced in varying quantities. Widely spaced geophysical transects show that rifting along some continental margins can transition from magma-poor to magma-rich. Our wide-angle seismic data from the Black Sea provide the first direct observations of such a transition. This transition coincides with a transform fault and is abrupt, occurring over only ~20–30 km. This abrupt transition cannot be explained solely by gradual along-margin variations in mantle properties, since these would be expected to result in a smooth transition from magma-poor to magma-rich rifting over hundreds of kilometers. We suggest that the abruptness of the transition results from the 3-D migration of magma into areas of greater extension during rifting, a phenomenon that has been observed in active rift environments such as mid-ocean ridges. (133 words)

6. The empirical data presented in this article reveal a segmented labor market and exploitation, with undocumented migrants not benefiting from international protection, human rights, nation state citizenship rights, or rights associated with the more recent concepts of postnational and transnational citizenship. (41 words)

다음 단락에서 사용된 연결어구를 나열한 뒤 이들이 왜 유용한지 설명하라. 부록2의 연습문제 해답에서 여러분의 답이 맞는지 확인해보라.

7. The systemic immune response in *Drosophila* is mediated by a battery of antimicrobial peptides produced largely by the fat body, an insect organ analogous to the mammalian liver. These peptides lyse microorganisms by forming pores in their cell walls. Functionally, the antimicrobial peptides fall into three classes depending on the pathogen specificity of their lytic activity. Thus, Drosomycin is a major antifungal peptide, whereas Diptericin is active against gram-negative bacteria, and Defensin works against gram-positive bacteria. Interestingly, infection of *Drosophila* with different classes of pathogens leads to preferential induction of the appropriate group of antimicrobial peptides.

다음 단락은 하이브리드 동물과 이들의 장기생존 및 생식에 관한 글이다. 이 글에 쉬운 영어의 원칙을 몇 가지나 적용할 수 있는가? 적용할 수 있는 원칙을 설명하라. 결과적으로 교정한 글이 간결해졌는가? 부록2의 연습문제 해답에서 여러분의 답이 맞는지 확인해보라.

8. Introgressive hybridization is most commonly observed in zones of geographical contact between otherwise allopatric taxa. Studies of such zones have provided important insights into the evolutionary process and have helped resolve part of the debate about fitness of hybrids. In many cases, most hybrid genotypes tend to be less fit than are the parental genotypes in parental habitats, owing either to endogenous or exogenous selection or both. However, theory predicts that some can be of equal or superior fitness in new habitats and, occasionally, even in parental habitats.

REFERENCE

1. Moore, R. *Writing to Learn Biology* (Saunders College Publishing, 1992).
2. Watson, J. D. & Crick, F. H. C. Molecular structure of nucleic acids. *Nature* **171**, 737–738 (1953).

제7장

오래된 정보와 새로운 정보

지금까지 우리는 명료하고 간결한 문장을 쉬운 영어로 쓰기 위한 원칙들, 즉 구체적인 주어와 강력한 능동태 동사, 불필요한 단어의 사용을 최소화하는 원칙들을 논했다. 하지만 글을 쓸 때 문장을 하나씩 따로 쓰지는 않는다. 우리는 문장을 묶어서 쓰며, 이러한 묶음이 단락을 형성한다. 이런 사실은 문장을 완전히 새로운 각도에서 생각하게 해준다. 실제로 문장에는 정해진 시작과 끝이 있으며, 독자는 그 각각에서 특정 정보를 찾고자 기대한다. 문장의 시작과 끝에 올바른 정보를 배치하면 독자의 기대를 충족시킬 수 있을 뿐 아니라 단락이 응집력을 갖게 된다.

| 오래된 정보는 문장의 앞부분에 두라

각 단락은 하나의 주인공 또는 아이디어를 중심으로 구성되어야 하며 그 주인공이 단락의 모든 문장의 주어가 되어야 한다. 독자는 이 주어에 익숙해지게 되고 이들 주어는 이제 오래된 정보로 인식된다. 대부분의 영어 문장에서는 주어가 동사 앞에 나오기 때문에 오래된 정보가 주어가 되면 독자는 문장의 앞부분에서 독자가 잘 아는 영역을 확보할 수 있다. 예를 들어 선형모델(linear models)에 관한 단락을 쓴다면 선형모델 또는 선형모델을 의미하는 단어들을 문장의 주어로 삼으라. 독자는 이런 주어를 볼 때마다 선형모델을 인식하게 될 것이고 여러분이 무엇을 말하고 있는지 알게 된다. 이렇게 되면 독자는 여러분이 주어(선형모델을 의미하는)에 대해 하고자 하는 말에 집중할 수 있게 된다. 아래의 좋은 예문을 살펴보자.

Quantum mechanics has enjoyed many successes since its formulation in the early 20th century. It has explained the structure and interactions of atoms, nuclei, and subnuclear particles, and has given rise to revolutionary technologies, such as integrated circuit chips and magnetic resonance imaging. At the same time, it has generated puzzles that persist to this day.

저자는 문장의 앞부분에 동일한 주인공을 지칭하는 일관적인 주어들을 사용했다: Quantum mechanics, It, it. 이 예문에서 볼 수 있듯이 일관적인 주어를 사용한다는 것이 동일한 단어를 사용한다는 의미는 아니다. 독자가 주어간의 연결고리를 쉽게 파악할 수 있다면 문제될 것이 없다.

| 새로운 정보를 문장의 뒷부분에 두라

오래되고 친숙한 정보를 문장의 앞부분에 두고 그 뒤에 강력한 동사를 배치하면 문장의 뒷부분에는 독자가 들어보지 못한 새로운 정보를 채울 수 있는 공간이 만들어진다. 좋은 농담의 펀치라인과 같이 바로 이 뒷부분이 스토리의 가장 흥미로운 부분이다. 독자는 문장의 뒷부분에 존재하는 정보에 주목하기 때문에 그 부분에 독자가 기억해주기 바라는 정보를 배치하라. 앞의 예문을 다시 살펴보자.

Quantum mechanics has enjoyed **many successes since its formulation in the early 20th century.** It has explained **the structure and interactions of atoms, nuclei, and subnuclear particles**, and has given rise **to revolutionary technologies, such as integrated circuit chips and magnetic resonance imaging.** At the same time, it has generated **puzzles that persist to this day.**

저자는 강력한 능동태의 동사를 주어 가까이에 두고 있다: has enjoyed, has explained, has generated. 두 번째 문장은 두 개의 절로 쪼개져 있으며, 각각 동사가 있다: has explained, has given rise. 모든 문장의 뒷부분(두 번째 문장의 경우 각절의 뒷부분)은 quantum mechanics에 관한 새로운 정보를 담고 있다: successes, uses(revolutionary technologies), puzzles.

물론 모든 단락에서 주어가 일관적으로 사용되는 것은 아니다. 위의 예문에서 저자는 독자가 quantum mechnics라는 주제에 익숙하리라고 생각했던 것 같다. 그래서 논문의 서론에 위치한 이 단락을 quantum mechanics에 관한 설명없이 시작하고 있다. 글의 주인공이 독자에게 익숙하지 않은 주제라면 한두 문장을 할애해서 설명돼 주인공을 독자가 가장 주목하기 좋은 장소, 곧 설명하는 문장의 뒷부분에 두라. 제3장에서 빌려온 아래의 좋은 예문을 살펴보자.

In the Great Lakes of Africa, large and diverse species **flocks of cichlid fish** have evolved rapidly. Lake Victoria, the largest of these lakes, had until recently at least 500 species of **haplochromine cichlids**. They were ecologically so diverse that they utilized almost all resources available to freshwater fishes in general, despite having evolved in perhaps as little as 12, 400 years and from a single ancestral species. This species **flock** is the most notable example of vertebrate explosive evolution known today. **Many** of its species have vanished within two decades, which can only partly be explained by predation by the introduced Nile perch (*Lates* spp.). Stenotopic rock-dwelling **cichlids**, of which there are more than 200 species, are rarely eaten by Nile perch. Yet, many such **species** have disappeared in the past 10 years.

저자는 주인공인 cichlid fish를 첫 두 문장의 뒷부분에 배치해서 소개하고 있다. 단락의 첫 문장은 In the Great Lakes of Africa라는 전치사구로 시작한다. 주어인 flocks와 전치사구인 of cichlid fish는 문장의 뒷부분에 등장한다. 주어인 Lake Victoria가 그 다음 문장을 시작하면 of의 목적어인 haplochromine cichlids는 문장의 마지막에 등장한다. 일단 독자가 익숙해지고 나면 cichlids 또는 이와 연관된 유사한 용어(they, flock, many, cichlids, species)가 나머지 문장의 앞부분에 주어로서 등장한다.

익숙하지 않은 주인공을 소개하는 경우 외에도 단락에서 주어를 바꿔야할 때가 있다. 동일한 방법을 사용하면 된다. 독자가 주목하는 장소인 문장의 마지막에 새로운 주인공을 도입한 다음 그 다음 문장의 주어로 새 주인공을 사용하라.

새 주인공을 문장 앞부분에서 소개하면 독자가 놀랜다. 그러기에 앞서서 새 주인 공을 그 앞 문장의 뒷부분에 소개함으로써 독자를 준비시키라. 다음에 좋은 예가 있다.

Supernovae deposit enormous amounts of energy into their surroundings. **They** play a key role in the heating of their host galaxies and in the enrichment of the interstellar medium with heavy elements that form the building blocks of life. Yet, the actual explosion **mechanism** is not well understood. One **way** to study the explosion is through the dynamics of the stellar debris that comprise supernova remnants such as **Cassiopeia A. Cas A** is the 2nd youngest known supernova remnant in the Galaxy (approximately 340 years old) and is also among the brightest. **It** is well studied at radio, X-ray, infrared, and optical wavelengths and is known to have two oppositely directed jets of ejecta with expansion velocities as high as 15, 000 km/s.

단락 전반부의 주인공인 supernovae는 첫 네 문장의 앞부분에서 주어로 활약한다: Supernovae, They, mechanism(explosion이 수식하고 있는), way(to study the explosion). 네 번째 문장의 뒷부분에는 새로운 주인공인 Cassiopeia A가 소개되며 따라서 우리는 새 주인공이 그 다음 두 문장의 새로운 주어로 등장할 때 준비가 되어있다: Cas A, It.

오래된 정보와 새로운 정보가 잘못 배치되는 것은 과학논문에서 흔히 일어나는 오류다. 그런 경우 흐름이 끊어지며 독자는 주요 논점을 놓치게 된다. 이런 오류가 일어나는 몇 가지 형태를 살펴보자.

❶ 오래된 정보를 문장의 뒷부분에 배치하는 경우가 있다. 이럴 경우 새로운 정보가 문장의 앞부분으로 밀려난다. 결과적으로 주요 논점이 담긴 새로운 정보가 독자가 기대하지 않는 위치에 놓인다. 말하고 싶은 논점을 결정하는 것은 저자의 몫이다. 하지만, 무엇을 말하고 싶던 간에 해당 정보는 문장의 뒷부분에 배치되어야한다. 다음 예문은 그렇지 않을 경우 어떤 문제가 일어나는지 잘 보여준다.

Wildland **fires** are disturbances that occur with long recurrence intervals and generally high severity in some forest types and with shorter intervals and lower severity in others. For millennia, wildland **fires** have arguably been the most important disturbance process throughout many western forests. Seed germination and establishment, growth patterns, plant community composition and structure, rates of mortality, soil productivity, and other properties and processes of western forest ecosystems are often strongly influenced and shaped by **fire disturbance regimes**. Even so, perhaps the most controversial aspect of western land management at present is the ecology of **fire and fire management**.

첫 두 문장에서는 주인공인 fires가 주어다. 이 오래된 정보 다음에는 이와 관련된 새로운 정보가 뒤따른다: 즉, 산불이 긴 또는 짧은 간격으로 발생하며 대다수의 서부 산림에서 가장 중요한 교란(disturbance)이라는 사실. 세 번째 문장은 새로운 정보인 germination and establishment를 갑작스럽게 문장 앞부분에, 오래된 정보인 fire disturbance regimes를 문장 뒷부분에 배치하고 있다. 네 번째 문장도 같은 오류를 범하고 있다. 산불이 controversial하다는 새로운 정보가 문장의 앞부분 근처에 등장하고 오래된 정보인 fire and fire management는 뒷부분에 나온다. 교정문에서는 일관적으로 fire가 문장 앞부분에 주어로 등장하고 산불이 중요한 이유와 산불이 controversial하다는 새로운 정보가 문장의 뒷부분에 배치되었다.

For millennia, wildland **fires** have been arguably the most important disturbances in many western forests. In some forest types, these **fires** occur infrequently with generally high severity, while in others, they occur frequently with lower severity. **Fire** strongly influences many aspects of western forest ecosystems including germination and establishment of seedlings, patterns of growth, composition, and structure of plant communities, rates of mortality, and productivity of soils. Even so, of the issues western land managers face, the ecology of **fire** and **fire management** are the most controversial.

❷ 오래된 정보가 문장의 뒷부분에 반복될 경우에도 오류가 일어난다.

Riparian forests in western North America <u>are</u> exceptionally important habitats and their ecological significance is often disproportionately important in relation to the amount of landscape they occupy. The <u>productivity</u> of **riparian habitats** <u>is</u> typically much higher than adjacent areas, and many species of plants and animals are restricted to **riparian habitats.** In areas of the arid west, **riparian** <u>forests</u> <u>constitute</u> less that 1% of the landscape, and yet well over 50% of the species of breeding birds depend on **those habitats.**

용어를 바꾸는 잘못 외에도 저자는 마지막 두 문장을 오래된 정보로 마치고 있다: riparian habitats, those habitats. 이것 때문에 새로운 정보가 독자가 주목하지 않는 문장의 중앙으로 밀려올라갔다. 오래된 정보를 이 두 문장의 뒷부분에서 제거해보자.

Riparian <u>forests</u> in western North America <u>are</u> exceptionally important. Although they occupy only a small part of the landscape, **they** <u>are</u> much more productive than adjacent areas, and many species of plants and animals are restricted to them. For example, in the arid west, **riparian** <u>forests</u> <u>constitute</u> less than 1% of the landscape, yet they support well over 50% of the breeding bird species.

❸ 새로운 정보를 새로운 정보가 소개되는 문장의 뒷부분이 아닌 앞부분에 두는 오류도 있다.

There <u>are</u> different **ways** in which international migrants can gain protection and/or rights. The <u>first</u> <u>is</u> the protection that exists for refugees under the terms of the 1951 Geneva Convention.

위 예문의 첫 문장을 살펴보면 앞으로 몇 문장에 걸쳐 발전될 정보는 바로 ways 이다. 하지만 ways는 문장의 앞부분에 주어로 등장한다. ways를 문장의 뒷부분에 배치하면 독자는 일련의 목록이 뒤따르리라 기대하게 된다.

International <u>migrants</u> <u>can gain</u> protection and/or rights in different **ways**. The <u>first</u> <u>is</u> the protection that exists for refugees under the terms of the 1951 Geneva Convention.

❹ 불필요한 단어가 문장의 뒷부분에 배치될 때도 있다. 이렇게 되면 새로운 정보 가 가려진다.

During my elementary school years, I <u>found</u> that my most exciting and rewarding moments came from the sense of wonder that I felt after learning something completely new **to me for the first time**. A second <u>wave</u> of amazement often <u>arrived</u> days or weeks later, when I actually began to understand **what I thought I had learned**.

저자는 이 예문에서 두 문장 모두의 뒷부분에 불필요한 단어들을 덧붙였다: to me for the first time은 new와 같은 의미이며, what I thought I had learned는 더 간 결하게 표현될 수 있다. 이런 단어들을 제거하면 주요 논점이 더욱 선명하게 드러 난다.

During my elementary school years, I <u>found</u> that my most exciting and rewarding moments came after learning something completely new. A second <u>wave</u> of amazement often <u>arrived</u> days or weeks later, when I actually began to understand it.

교정된 두 번째 문장 끝에 대명사 it을 두었다는 점에 주목하라. 문장 뒷부분에 서 불필요한 단어나 어구를 대명사로 대치할 경우 대명사의 바로 앞 단어가 강조 되며 이 경우에는 understand에 힘이 실린다.

❶ 다음의 문장 및 단락에서 저자는 오래된 정보와 새로운 정보를 올바른 위치에 배치하고 있는가? 우리가 논의한 원칙들을 이용해서 잘못된 문장을 교정하라. 부록2의 연습문제 해답에서 여러분의 답이 맞는지 확인해보라.

1. Unfortunately, as noted 40 years ago, few students experience the thrill of doing field science because they are rarely allowed to leave the confines of the classroom to become immersed in field-based science.

2. Bank erosion rates along the South River in Virginia increased by factors of 2–3 after 1957. Increased bank erosion rates cannot be explained by changes in the intensity of either freeze-thaw or storm intensity, and changes in the density of riparian trees should have decreased erosion rates.

3. Students majoring in science often believe they can escape the intensive writing and presentations that their peers in the humanities and social sciences must do. However, science is a collective human endeavor whose success hinges upon effective communication, both written and oral. Even if findings are ground breaking, they are potentially worthless if they can't be shared with others in a clear and engaging way. Teaching undergraduate science students to effectively communicate is therefore an essential goal.

4. Climate plays an important part in determining the average numbers of a species, and periodical seasons of extreme cold or drought, I believe to be the most effective of all checks. I estimated that the winter of 1854–55 destroyed four-fifths of the birds in my own grounds; and this is a tremendous destruction, when we remember that ten per cent is an extraordinarily severe mortality from epidemics with man. The action of climate seems at first sight to be quite independent of the struggle for existence; but in so far as climate chiefly acts in reducing food, it brings on the most severe struggle between the individuals, whether of the same or of distinct species, which subsist on the same kind of food. Even when climate, for instance extreme cold, acts directly, it will be the least vigorous, or those which have got least food through the advancing winter, which will suffer most.

제8장

목록을 나열할 때는 평행구조로

때로는 한 문장에서 하나 이상의 새로운 정보를 독자에게 전달하는 경우가 있다. 구조가 평행을 이루면 두 개 이상의 정보를 더 쉽게 읽을 수 있다. 평행구조란 어떤 목록의 아이템을 비슷한 문법적 구조 안에서 유사한 단어를 가지고 나열하는 방식을 말한다. 다음의 좋은 예를 살펴보자.

A successful phenomenology must accomplish many things: **it must explain** why repetitions of the same measurement lead to definite, but differing, outcomes, **and** why the probability distribution of outcomes is given by the Born rule; **it must permit** quantum coherence to be maintained for atomic and mesoscopic systems, **while** predicting definite outcomes for measurements with realistic apparatus sizes in realistic measurement times; **it should conserve** overall probability, **so** that particles do not spontaneously disappear; and **it should not allow** superluminal transmission of signals.

위 예문에서 소개된 목록의 아이템을 살펴보면 각각이 얼마나 유사한 방식으로 묘사되었는지 알 수 있다:

it must explain ⋯, and
it must permit ⋯, while

it should conserve …, so

and it should not allow …

각 아이템은 독립절에서 it이라는 일관적인 주어로 시작되며 그 뒤에는 조동사 인 must 또는 should가, 그 다음에는 능동형 동사인 explain, permit, conserve, allow 가 뒤따른다. 처음 세 개의 독립절은 접속사 and, while, so로 시작하는 의존절을 포함하고 있다. 단락의 마지막 문장에는 종속절이 없지만 앞에서 반복되어온 리 듬이 유지된다.

다음 예문은 평행구조를 갖고 있지 않다.

These similarities include an early sensitive period, an innate filtering mechanism that isolates conspecific vocalizations, a babbling developmental phase, and the importance of social variables in vocal learning.

이 문장은 새가 노래하는 법을 배울 때 거치는 네 단계를 나열하고 있다. 각 단 계가 하나의 어구로 설명되지만 구마다 형태가 상이하기 때문에 목록을 읽고 기 억하기가 어렵다. 이 단락의 목록에 포함된 아이템은 다음과 같다.

an early sensitive period,

an innate filtering mechanism that isolates conspecific vocalizations,

a babbling development phase, and

the importance of social variables in vocal learning.

첫 번째 어구는 부정관사 an으로 시작되고 두 개의 형용사(early, sensitive) 가 나온 뒤에 명사인 period가 뒤따른다. 이 패턴은 세 번째 어구(a babbling developmental phase)에서도 반복되지만 두 번째 및 네 번째 어구에서는 패턴이 바 뀐다. 두 번째 어구도 비슷한 방식으로 시작되지만(an innate filtering mechanism) 종속절을 포함하고 있다(that isolates conspecific vocalizations). 네 번째 어구는 부 정관사가 아닌 정관사 the로 시작되며 추상명사인 importance와 두 개의 전치사구 인 of social variables와 in vocal learning이 뒤따른다.

이 목록을 평행구조로 만들려면 각 어구를 동일한 방식으로 구조화해야 한다. 나는 두 번째 어구의 종속절인 that isolates conspecific vocalizations를 제거했으며 저자가 이 내용을 나중에 자세히 언급할 수 있으리라 믿는다. 또한 주인공을 설명하기 위해서 하나의 용어를 선택했다. 원문에는 세 개의 주인공이 등장한다: period, mechanism, phase. 교정문의 목록은 다음과 같다:

an early sensitive phase,
a filtering phase,
a babbling phase,
a social phase.

이제 모든 아이템이 평행구조를 갖는다.

These similarities include **an early sensitive phase, a filtering phase, a babbling phase, and a social phase.**

연습문제

⓬ 아래 문장이 제공하는 목록을 주의깊게 살펴보라. 평행구조를 가지고 있는가? 우리가 논의한 원칙들을 이용해서 잘못된 문장을 교정하라. 부록2의 연습문제 해답에서 여러분의 답이 맞는지 확인해보라.

1. Central to this deficit has been the rising average age of the nursing workforce and the decline in the number of hours worked; fewer nurses are working standard full-time hours (35-44 hours per week) and 44 percent work part-time.

2. The problem of finding the optimal strokes of hypothetical microswimmers has drawn a lot of attention in recent years. Problems that have been solved include the optimal stroke pattern of Purcell's three-link swimmer, an ideal elastic flagellum, a shape-changing body, a two- and a three-sphere swimmer, and a spherical squirmer.

3. Cilia are hair-like protrusions that beat in an asymmetric fashion to pump the fluid in the direction of their effective stroke. They propel certain protozoa, such as *Paramecium*, and also fulfill a number of functions in mammals, including mucous clearance from airways, left–right asymmetry determination, and transport of an egg cell in fallopian tubes.

4. Integrons consist of three elements: an attachment site where the horizontally acquired sequence is integrated; a gene encoding a site-specific recombinase (that is, integrase); and a promoter that drives expression of the incorporated sequence.

5. North American (NA)-EEEV strains cause periodic outbreaks of mosquito-borne encephalitis in humans and equines, are highly neurovirulent, and, in comparison with related Venezuelan equine encephalitis virus (VEEV) and western equine encephalitis virus (WEEV), cause far more severe encephalitic disease in humans.

제**9**장
문장의 길이에 변화를 주라

좋은 글은 다양한 길이의 문장으로 구성된다. 긴 문장(30단어 이상)은 읽기가 어렵고, 짧은 문장(10단어 이하)은 졸렬해 보이며, 중간 길이의 문장(15-25단어)은 단조롭게 느껴진다. 과학논문의 저자가 짧은 문장을 남용했다고 비판받는 경우는 드물다. 과학논문의 저자는 흔히 중간 길이 문장 및 긴 문장을 사용하며 비슷한 문장 길이를 논문 전체에 걸쳐 유지한다. 다음 예를 살펴보자.

One of the major goals of conservation biology is to conduct scientific research that will aid in the preservation of natural landscapes. (22 words) Of particular concern to scientists and environmentalists are natural areas that have remained relatively undisturbed for long periods of time. (20 words) These areas often serve as habitats for a variety of plant and animal species that are not found in more disturbed areas. (22 words) Accordingly, these lands are often set aside as protected areas. (10 words) These areas, although protected from urbanization and development, are often subject to high levels of disturbance from recreational activities. (19 words) Thus, land managers must struggle to find an acceptable balance between biological and social management objectives. (16 words)

이 글은 여러 측면에서 찬사를 받을 만하다: 주어가 구체적이고 동사는 대부분

능동태이다(추상명사가 남용되면서 대부분 약한 동사이기는 하지만). 주어와 동사는 가까이 배치되어 있으며 오래된 정보와 새로운 정보도 올바르게 배치되어 있다. 하지만, 거의 모든 문장의 길이가 비슷하고(16-22단어) 이로 인해 글이 수면제 수준으로 단조롭다. 일부 문장은 묶고 일부 문장은 길이를 줄임으로써 문장의 길이에 변화를 주면 독자의 관심을 끄는 데 도움이 된다.

Conservation biologists strive to preserve natural landscapes. (7 words) They are particularly concerned with areas that have a long history of protection where a variety of plants and animals can be found that are absent from more disturbed areas. (30 words) Often however, these areas are subject to high levels of disturbance from recreational activities. (14 words) By providing quantitative data on the effects of recreation on the surrounding biota, conservation biologists can help land mangers find a balance between social and biological demands. (27 words)

　위의 교정문에서는 문장의 길이가 7단어(짧은 문장)에서 14-27단어(중간 길이), 30단어(긴 문장)에 이른다. 그 결과 글을 더욱 흥미롭게 읽을 수 있다.
　다음에 나오는 잘 쓰여진 예문에서는 문장의 길이가 11단어에서 26단어를 넘나든다. 첫 문장과 마지막 문장은 대시 기호로 나뉘어져 있으며 따라서 각 문장이 두 개의 짧은 문장으로 이루어져 있다는 인상을 준다: 첫 문장은 4단어와 7단어의 문장, 마지막 문장은 6단어와 10단어의 문장. 짧은 문장은 결정적인 펀치를 날리면서 주요 논점을 강조할 수 있고 긴 문장은 리듬을 더해준다는 점에 주목하라. 글에는 이 두 요소가 적절히 배합되어야 한다.

Most nematodes are gonochoristic—they produce XO males and XX females. (11 words) The males make small, round spermatids that activate following mating, extend pseudopods, and crawl toward the spermathecae of the female, where they compete to fertilize oocytes. (26 words) However, some species have evolved an androdioecious mating system, with XO males and self-fertile XX hermaphrodites. (16 words) In these species, the hermaphrodites make spermatids late in larval development and then permanently switch to the production of oocytes. (20 words) In almost all respects, the male and hermaphrodite sperm from these species appear identical. (14 words) However, one trait is sexually dimorphic—the male sperm are much larger than those of hermaphrodites. (16 words)

이 예문에 등장하는 문장의 평균 길이는 18단어이며 이는 추천되는 문장 길이의 상한선인 20-25단어보다 짧다. 문장의 평균길이를 이 상한선보다 낮게 유지하면 아래 예문과 같이 긴 문장의 남용을 막을 수 있다.

Further processing [of the heterodimer] to generate an intracellular fragment able to traverse to the nucleus was dependent upon ligand binding, resulting in casein kinase-dependent phosphorylation followed by enzymic cleavage likely involving an ADAM (a disintegrin and metalloprotease) type metalloprotease sequentially followed by further intracytoplasmic cleavage by the γ-secretase complex. (49 words)

이 문장은 너무 길다. 내용이 복잡하다는 점을 생각해보면 더욱 그러하다. 교정하려면 일련의 액션을 쪼개서 각 액션을 하나의 문장에 담으라. 긴 문장은 대개 하나 이상의 논점을 갖고 있으며 이를 쪼개면 의미가 더욱 분명해진다.

Further processing of the heterodimer to generate an intracellular fragment able to traverse to the nucleus was dependent upon ligand binding, resulting in casein kinase-dependent phosphorylation. (26 words) This was followed by enzymic cleavage likely involving an ADAM (a disintegrin and metalloprotease) type metalloprotease. (16 words) The product was then cleaved by the γ-secretase complex. (12 words)

교정문에서는 각 단계가 짧은 문장으로 전달되며 따라서 독자가 쉽게 따라갈 수 있다.

연습문제

⑬ 아래 문장의 단어 수를 카운트하라. 문장 길이가 다양한가? 문장 당 평균 단어수는 몇인가? 평균이 짧은가 아니면 긴가? 문장 길이를 개선하기 위한 여러분의 제안은 무엇인가? 예를 들어보라. 부록2의 연습문제 해답에서 여러분의 답이 맞는지 확인해보라.

1. In order to unravel the mode of action of neuronal networks, a neurobiologist's dream would be not only to be able to monitor neuronal activity but also to have control over distinct sets of neurons and to be able to manipulate their activity and observe the effect on behavior. This idea is not new. As the activity of a neuron is based on the depolarization of its cell membrane, neuronal activity can be induced by an experimenter using stimulation electrodes by which the cell membrane can be artificially depolarized or hyperpolarized. Although stimulation electrodes have served, and continue to serve, neuroscientists well for decades, limitations of this invasive approach are obvious.

다음의 긴 문장을 짧은 문장들로 나누라.

2. The extrapolation from *in vitro* measurements to the *in vivo* behavior of proteins is hampered by extremely high (300–400mg/mL) intracellular macromolecular concentrations in the cell, i.e. crowding, which is one of the most important factors that influences the structure and function of proteins under physiological conditions. (47 words)

3. Some of the confusion about the role of hybridization in evolutionary diversification stems from the contradiction between a perceived necessity for cessation of gene flow to enable adaptive population differentiation on the one hand, and the potential of hybridization for generating adaptive variation, functional novelty, and new species on the other. (52 words)

제10장
단락을 디자인하라

이제 초점을 문장 수준의 교정이 아닌 단락의 디자인으로 바꾸어보자. 단락도 문장과 마찬가지로 특정 구성요소를 지니고 있으며(이슈, 발전, 결론, 요점) 독자는 각 구성요소에서 특정 정보를 기대한다. 독자는 단락을 읽어나갈 때 이런 구성요소에 의지해 새로운 아이디어를 인식하고 이를 뒷받침하는 증거를 수집 및 재해석한다. 구성요소 중 어느 하나라도 빠져 있거나 정보가 잘못 배치되어 있다면 독자는 혼란에 빠지게 된다. 이번 장에서는 서로 다른 두 종류의 단락을 이용해 각 구성요소를 설명할 것이다. 한 단락은 논문이 시작할 때 등장하는 서론 단락이고, 다른 하나는 논문의 나머지 부분을 이루는 본론 단락이다.

우선, 길이에 관해 몇 마디 덧붙이고자 한다. 논문의 단락 하나를 읽기 시작하는 독자를 상상해보자. 빽빽한 글이 긴 블록을 차지하고 있으면 독자의 기가 꺾인다. 단락의 단어수를 카운트해서 단어수가 200을 넘으면 나누라. 이상적인 단락은 약 150개의 단어로 구성되며 물론 경우에 따라 조금씩 달라진다.

| 이슈(Issue)

각 단락은 독자에게 이 단락의 주제가 무엇인지 알림으로써 시작되어야 한다. 우리는 이를 주제문(a topic sentence)이라 부르지만 훌륭한 저자들이 두세 개의 문장으로 단락을 시작하는 경우도 있기 때문에 단수형의 주제문이라는 용어가 혼란을 줄 수 있다. 주제문보다 더 좋은 용어는 바로 이슈이다. 길이에 상관없이 이슈는 단락의 나머지 부분에서 상세히 다루어질 주인공과 액션을 소개하는 것으로 끝나야 한다. 아래 단락에서는 이슈가 한 문장으로 제기되고 있다.

Determining the cause of HIV-1 resistance in Old World monkey cells stymied HIV researchers for nearly two decades. An early view was that the block resulted from expression of an incompatible receptor on the surface of Old World monkey cells. However, identification of the HIV-1 co-receptor in the mid-1990s disproved this hypothesis. Subsequent studies demonstrated that HIV-1 could enter Old World monkey cells, but a block that targeted the viral capsid prevented the establishment of a permanent infection.

이 예문의 이슈인 첫 문장은 저자가 단락의 나머지 부분에서 발전시키고자 하는 주요 논점을 요약해준다: how Old World monkey's resistance to HIV-1 has stymied researchers for two decades. 또한, 이슈는 단락의 주인공과 액션을 소개하고 있다: HIV-1, Old World monkeys, stymied, researchers.

다음 예문의 이슈는 두 문장으로 되어 있다.

We initially hypothesized that TRIM5α functioned as a cofactor necessary for capsid uncoating. However, subsequent findings argued against this hypothesis. First, knocking down human TRIM5α showed no effects on HIV-1 replication in human cells. Second, rodent cells, which do not express TRIM5α, supported HIV-1 infection if engineered to express an appropriate receptor. Finally, human TRIM5α does not associate with the HIV-1 capsid in biochemical assays. Thus, TRIM5α appeared to have evolved primarily as an inhibitory factor aimed at thwarting viral replication, rather than a host factor co-opted by HIV-1 to promote infection.

저자는 첫 문장에서 하나의 가설을 제시하고 두 번째 문장에서는 이를 기각한다. 단락의 나머지에서는 해당 가설을 기각시킨 연구결과를 설명한다. 단락의 나머지에서 발전시킬 주인공과 액션은 이슈의 거의 마지막에서 소개된다: subsequent findings, argued.

| 발전(Development)

단락의 앞부분에서 이슈를 제기한 다음 저자가 이를 확장시키는 것을 발전이라 부른다. 발전을 잘 쓰는 방법 중 하나는 앞 예문의 저자가 한 바와 같이 어떤 결론으로 이끄는 잘 정의된 단계들을 설명하는 것이다.

We initially hypothesized that TRIM5α functioned as a cofactor necessary for capsid uncoating. However, subsequent findings argued against this hypothesis. **First, knocking down human TRIM5α showed no effects on HIV-1 replication in human cells. Second, rodent cells, which do not express TRIM5α, supported HIV-1 infection if engineered to express an appropriate receptor. Finally, human TRIM5α does not associate with the HIV-1 capsid in biochemical assays.** Thus, TRIM5α appeared to have evolved primarily as an inhibitory factor aimed at thwarting viral replication, rather than a host factor co-opted by HIV-1 to promote infection.

이 예문의 발전은 세 문장으로 구성되어 있으며 각 문장은 연결어구로 시작되기 때문에 독자가 정보를 따라가는 것을 도와준다: First, Second, Finally.

이슈를 발전시키는 다른 방법은 예를 들거나 전문가의 의견을 제시하는 것이다. 또는 이슈에 어떻게든 자격을 부여할 수도 있다. 때로는 이슈가 하나의 질문으로 제기되며 저자는 발전을 이용해 이슈에 답할 수 있다.

Does TRIM5α have the ability to block infection by other retroviruses? **We found that TRIM5α from various Old World monkey species conferred potent resistance to HIV-1, but not SIV. New World monkey TRIM5α proteins, in contrast, blocked SIV but not HIV-1 infection. Human TRIM5α inhibited N-MLV and EIAV replication.** Thus the variation among TRIM5 orthologs accounts for the observed patterns of post-entry blocks to retroviral replication among primate species.

이 예문의 발전은 이슈에서 제기된 질문에 답하고 있으며 다음을 설명하는 세 문장으로 구성되어 있다: TRIM5α's ability to block infection in Old World monkeys, New World monkeys, humans.

| 결론(Conclusion)

독자는 단락에서 새로운 개념이 소개되고 발전된 후에는 단락의 마지막에서 일종의 독해 점검 역할을 하는 문장을 찾는다 – 내가 저자의 의도를 잘 이해했나? 이 마지막 문장, 즉 결론은 독자에게 생각할 여지를 준다. 다음 단락에서 새로운 개념을 소개하기 전에 독자에게 생각할 시간을 선사하라. 다음의 두 연속된 단락을 살펴보자.

Does TRIM5α have the ability to block infection by other retroviruses? We found that TRIM5α from various Old World monkey species conferred potent resistance to HIV-1, but not SIV. New World monkey TRIM5α proteins, in contrast, blocked SIV but not HIV-1 infection. Human TRIM5α inhibited N-MLV and EIAV replication. **Thus the variation among TRIM5 orthologs accounts for the observed patterns of post-entry blocks to retroviral replication among primate species.**

To determine why Old World monkey TRIM5α, but not human TRIM5α, potently blocks HIV-1, we systematically altered the human sequence to more closely resemble the monkey sequence. Remarkably, we found that a single amino acid determines the antiviral potency of human TRIM5α. If a positively charged arginine residue in the C-terminal domain of human TRIM5α is either deleted or replaced with an uncharged amino acid, human cells gain the ability to inhibit HIV-1 infection. **Perhaps some humans have already acquired this change and are naturally resistant to HIV-1 infection.**

첫 단락의 결론은 이슈에서 제기된 질문에 관한 대답을 요약하고 있다. 요약은 결론의 흔한 형태다. 이 예문에서는 발전에서 확장된 정보를 재구성해서 좀더 넓은 문맥으로 제시하고 있다. 이제 독자는 다음 사실을 확실히 알게된다: **TRIM5 α blocks infection by other retroviruses**. 따라서, 두 번째 단락의 이슈에서 제기되는 새로운 질문을 공략할 준비가 되어 있다: why does Old World monkey TRIM5α, but not human TRIM5α, block HIV-1?

위 예문의 두 번째 단락 마지막 문장은 결론을 쓰는 또 다른 방법을 보여준다. 질문을 던지거나 이유를 추측하는 것은 발전을 자연스럽게 확장하는 일이다. 이런 식의 결론은 독자에게 생각할 여지를 남겨준다.

단락의 결론을 내리는 방식은 여러 가지다. 하지만 다음 단락에 속하는 이슈를 언급하는 일은 피해야 한다. 단락의 결론은 요약하고 추측하거나 앞의 정보를 소화한 독자에게 질문을 던지는 곳이지 친숙하지 않은 내용으로 독자를 놀라게 하는 곳이 아니다. 이슈는 새로운 단락의 앞부분을 위해 남겨두라.

┃ 논제(Point)

우리는 지금까지 본론 단락의 이슈, 발전, 결론을 다루었다. 하지만, 서론 단락에서는 이런 기본 바탕을 한 가지 중요한 방식으로 변형해야 한다. 서론은 논문 전체를 기준으로 보면 이슈에 해당하지만, 논문의 길이에 따라 세 개 또는 그 이상의 단락으로 구성될 수 있다. 길이가 얼마가 되건 상관없이 서론의 마지막 단락의 끝에는 앞으로 나올 글 전체를 예견하는 문장 하나가 있어야 한다. 전통적으로는 이를 테제(thesis)라고 불렀지만 이 단어는 과학 분야에서 다른 뜻으로 널리 사용되기 때문에 혼란을 피할 수 있는 논제(point)가 더 좋은 용어다. 논제는 앞으로 벌어질 일에 대해 독자를 준비시켜 주기 때문에 중요하다. 논제가 없으면 혼란이 야기된다. 다음 예문은 상을 받은 과학논문의 서론이며 나는 이번 장의 모든 예문을 이 논문에서 발췌했다.[1] 논제를 찾아보라.

Humans have been exposed to retroviruses for millions of years. Indeed, a significant portion of our genome consists of endogenous retroviruses—reminders of our vulnerability to past infections. The HIV/AIDS epidemic, which began nearly a century ago when simian immunodeficiency virus (SIV) passed from chimpanzees into a human host, is the latest episode in the longstanding coevolutionary struggle between retroviruses and their hosts.

Human immunodeficiency virus type 1 (HIV-1) causes AIDS in humans, and to a lesser extent, in chimpanzees. However, not long after the discovery of HIV-1, scientists realized that certain primate species were resistant to HIV-1 infection. In particular, monkeys from Africa and Asia, referred to as Old World monkeys, could not be infected with HIV-1 and did not develop AIDS. This discovery brought both excitement and frustration. The block to HIV-1 replication in Old World monkey cells hindered efforts to develop an animal model for testing drugs and vaccines. On the other hand, Old World monkeys had evolved for millions of years in Africa—the epicenter of the current HIV-1 epidemic. Perhaps exposure to past HIV-1–like epidemics led to the emergence of an antiviral defense that protects them against HIV-1.

논제는 앞으로 일어날 바를 예견해주는 문장이며 이 예문에서는 두 번째 단락의 끝에 위치한다. 이 문장을 통해 우리는 논문의 나머지에서 발전될 주제를 알게 된다: an antiviral defense that protects Old World monkeys from HIV-1 infection.

연습문제

⑭ 다음의 본문 단락에서 이슈를 찾아라. 저자는 이슈를 어떻게 발전시키고 있는가? 부록2의 연습문제 해답에서 여러분의 답이 맞는지 확인해보라.

1. Males of *O. acuminatus* [dung beetles] employed two very different tactics to encounter and mate with females: they either attempted to monopolize access to a female by guarding the entrance to her tunnel (guarding), or they attempted to bypass guarding males (sneaking). Guarding behavior entailed remaining inside a tunnel with a female, and fighting intruding males over possession of the tunnel. Guarding males blocked tunnel entrances and periodically "patrolled" the length of the tunnel. Rival males could gain possession of a tunnel only by forcibly evicting the resident male, and both fights and turnovers were frequent. Fights over tunnel occupancy entailed repeated butting, wrestling and pushing of opponents, and fights continued

until one of the contestants left the tunnel.

2. One prerequisite for the maintenance of dimorphism is that organisms experience a fitness tradeoff across environments. If animals encounter several discrete environment types, or ecological or behavioral situations, and these different environments favor different morphologies, then distinct morphological alternatives can evolve within a single population—each specialized for one of the different environments. Such fitness tradeoffs have been demonstrated for several dimorphic species. For example, soft and hard seed diets have favored two divergent bill morphologies within populations of African finches, and high and low levels of predation have favored alternative shell morphologies in barnacles, and spined and spineless morphologies in rotifers and *Daphnia*. It is possible that the alternative reproductive tactics characterized in this study produce a similar situation in *O. acuminatus*. If guarding and sneaking behaviors favor horned and hornless male morphologies, respectively, then the reproductive behavior of males may have contributed to the evolution of male horn length dimorphism in this species.

3. In recent times, the origin of the adaptive immune response has been uncovered. It turns out that the two recombinase-activated genes are encoded in a short stretch of DNA, in opposite orientations and lacking exons. This suggested an origin in a retroposon, as did the presence of the recognition signal sequences that lie 3' of all V gene segments and 5' of all J gene segments. This hypothesis was tested *in vitro* and shown to be true. Other processes expand diversity tremendously, such as the generation of D gene segments in the first chain to rearrange, the nucleotide-adding enzyme TdT that inserts nucleotides in the junctions of V-D-J junctions, and somatic hypermutation.

다음의 각 단락에서 이슈와 발전, 결론이 무엇인지 설명하라.

4. Despite a consistent correlation between genome size and the obligate association with host cells, genome reduction is not simply an adaptive response to living within hosts. Instead, the trend toward large-scale gene loss reflects a lack of effective selection for maintaining genes in these specialized

microbes. Because the host presents a constant environment rich in metabolic intermediates, some genes are rendered useless by adoption of a strictly symbiotic or pathogenic life-style. These superfluous sequences are eliminated through mutational bias favoring deletions, a process apparently universal in bacterial lineages. Thus, all of the fully sequenced small genomes display a pattern of loss of biosynthetic pathways, such as those for amino acids that can be obtained from the host cytoplasm.

5. Unlike pathogens, symbionts may devote part of their genomes to processes that are more directly beneficial to the host rather than to the bacterial cell itself. *Buchnera* retains and even amplifies genes for the biosynthesis of amino acids required by hosts, devoting almost 10% of its genome to these pathways, which are missing from pathogens with similarly small genomes. Because of their fastidious growth requirements, the biological role of obligately associated symbionts can rarely be determined experimentally. However, genome comparisons can provide a means for determining their functions in hosts. Such future research should reveal, for example, whether the endosymbionts of blood-feeding hosts, such as *Wigglesworthia glossinia* in tsetse flies, retain pathways for biosynthesis of vitamins absent from blood, whether the symbiont *Vibrio fischeri* provides functions other than bioluminescence to its squid host, and whether the mutualistic *Wolbachia* of filarial nematodes contain genes for host benefit that are absent in the parasitic *Wolbachia* of arthropods.

─── REFERENCE ─────────────────────────────────

1. Stremlau, M. Why Old World Monkeys are resistant to HIV-1. *Science* **318**, 1565–1566 (2007).

제11장
단락을 재배열하라

　단락의 디자인 교정을 마칠 즈음이 되면 일부를 재배열할 필요가 있다. 좋은 저자는 독자가 논문 전체를 쉽게 항해하면서 주요 논점을 이해할 수 있도록, 예측 가능한 패턴으로 단락을 배열한다.

　대개는 한 논문에서 여러 개의 단락 배열 패턴이 나타난다. 이런 패턴은 한 단락 내에서 문장을 배열할 때 사용되기도 하며, 특별히 많은 정보를 담고 있는 단락의 경우 그러하다.

| 시간적 순서

　과학연구는 하나의 프로세스, 즉 어떤 결과를 도출하기 위해 이루어지는 연관된 액션들의 연속이다. 예를 들어, 하나의 실험은 여러 단계를 포함하며, 각 단계는 특정한 순서대로 이루어진다. 또한, 특정 생화학적 경로는 일련의 여러 생화학적 반응으로 이루어진다. 이런 정보를 전달하는 가장 논리적인 방법은 시간적 순서를 따르는 것이다. 일단 순서가 정해지면 논문 전체에 걸쳐 동일한 순서를 유지하라. 말똥풍뎅이(dung beetles)에 관한 논문의 방법 섹션에서 발췌한 좋은 예문을 살펴보자.

To compare the reproductive behaviors of horned and hornless males, I observed their methods of mate-acquisition both without and with competition from a rival male. **In the first experiment**, one male and one female were placed in each of 12 observation chambers. Seven of these males were hornless, five were horned, and females were selected at random. Beetles were observed for a minimum of three half- hour intervals (maximum of six intervals), during which time all behaviors were recorded.

In the second experiment, two males (one horned and one hornless) were placed together in each observation chamber with a single female, and behaviors of all individuals were monitored as above. This second experiment tested for behavioral differences arising as a result of direct competition for access to females. Because dung always had large numbers of *O. acuminatus*, and because horned and hornless males occurred in approximately equal frequencies on Barro Colorado Island, this experiment accurately reflected natural conditions experienced by males.

저자는 각 실험을 시간적 순서에 따라 설명하는 방식으로 단락을 배열했다. 결과 섹션에서도 동일한 순서가 유지된다. 실험1의 결과가 기술되고, 그 다음에 실험2의 결과가 나오는 순으로. 물론 실험이 항상 단선적으로만 진행되는 것은 아니다. 실험결과에 따라 처음의 가설을 바꾸고 다시 시작해야 할 수도 있다. 그럴 경우 실험을 시간적 순서에 따라 보고할 수 없게 된다. 이런 경우 스토리가 논리적이 되도록 실험을 배열하라.

단락을 시간적 순서로 배열하는 것은 어떤 프로세스를 설명할 때 효과적이다. 하지만, 과학논문은 다른 패턴의 단락 배열이 요구되는 많은 종류의 정보로 이루어져 있다.

일반적인 내용에서 구체적인 내용으로

모든 스토리에는 서론이 있다. 예를 들어 과학논문의 서론은 익숙하지 않은 주제를 이해하는 데 필요한 배경지식을 독자에게 제공해준다. 익숙하지 않은 정보를 전달할 때 사용되는 논리적 방법 중 하나는 일반적인 내용에서 구체적인 내용으로 진행하는 것이다. 첫 단락에서는 해당 주제에 관한 일반적인 개론을 제시하고 이어지는 단락에서는 논문의 구체적인 초점에 이를 때까지 주제를 점점 좁혀나가는 것이다. 다음의 좋은 예를 살펴보자.

Predation is a major cause of mortality for most species of animals, and many produce **alarm calls** when they perceive a potential predator. **Alarm calls** often differ in acoustic structure, depending on the situation in which they are produced. If a species is preyed upon by different predators that use different hunting strategies or vary in the degree of danger they present, selection can favor variation in alarm calls that encode this information. **Such variation in alarm calls** can be used to transfer information about the type of predator, the degree of threat that a predator represents, or both.

In addition to discriminating among broad types of predators (e.g., raptor versus snake), discriminating among morphologically similar predators within a single type (e.g., different species of raptors) could also be adaptive if the predators vary in the degree of threat they pose. One species that is faced with numerous, morphologically similar predators is the **black-capped chickadee** (*Poecile atricapilla*). Chickadees are small, common songbirds that are widespread throughout North America. In the non-breeding season, chickadees form flocks of six to eight birds. **They use an elaborate system of vocalizations** to mediate social interactions in these flocks and **to warn conspecifics about predators.**

첫 문장에서 저자는 많은 동물이 잡혀먹는 것을 피하기 위해 경보음(alarm calls)을 사용한다고 소개한다. 그런 다음 서로 다른 종류의 포식자에 관한 정보를 담은 다양한 경보음을 소개한다. 두 번째 단락이 끝날 즈음에 저자는 경보음을 이용해 비슷한 종류의 포식자를 구별할 수 있는 특별한 동물, the black-capped chickadee

를 소개한다.

과학논문의 고찰(discussion)에서는 이와는 정반대의 배열, 즉 구체적인 발견에서 시작해서 일반적인 의미로 진행하는 방식이 통상적으로 사용된다. 다음에 좋은 예가 있다.

In total, our results show that the introduction of foxes to the Aleutian archipelago transformed the islands from grasslands to maritime tundra. Fox predation reduced seabird abundance and distribution, in turn reducing nutrient transport from sea to land. The more nutrient-impoverished ecosystem that resulted favored less productive forbs and shrubs over more productive grasses and sedges.

These findings have several broad implications. First, they show that strong direct effects of introduced predators on their naive prey can ultimately have dramatic indirect effects on entire ecosystems and that these effects may occur over large areas — in this case across an entire archipelago. Second, they bolster growing evidence that the flow of nutrients, energy, and material from one ecosystem to another can subsidize populations and, importantly, influence the structure of food webs. Finally, they show that the mechanisms by which predators exert ecosystem-level effects extend beyond both the original conceptual model provided by Hairston *et al.* and its more recent elaborations.

첫 단락에서 저자는 실험의 구체적인 결과를 요약하고 있다. 두 번째 단락은 더 일반적인 내용을 담고 있으며 실험결과의 의미를 확장해 설명한다.

| 가장 덜 중요한 내용에서 가장 중요한 내용으로

과학논문의 목적 중 한 가지는 설득하는 것이다. 가장 덜 중요한 증거에서 가장 중요한 증거로 이동하는 패턴의 배열은 글에 설득력을 더해준다. 중요한 개념을 글의 뒷부분에 두면 더 설득력이 생기는 것은 문장의 뒷부분에 새롭고 중요한 정보를 배치했을 때 독자가 더 잘 기억하는 것과 같은 이치다. 이 원칙은 새로운 정보가 문장의 뒷부분에 있건, 한 단락의 뒷부분에 있건, 아니면 일군의 단락의 뒷부분에 있건 동일하다. 책의 어느 한 장(章)의 서론에서 발췌한 다음 글을 살펴보자.

Many species of crustaceans have enlarged appendages used in fighting. In stomatopods, for example, the second pair of maxillipeds has been lengthened and strengthened to produce powerful weapons, the "raptorial appendages," which are used in both prey capture and fighting (figure 4.5). A subset of the stomatopods, species termed "smashers," use their raptorial appendages to disable armored prey such as mollusks and crabs. When these weapons are used against conspecifics, they are capable of causing serious injury, even death. In another group, the snapping shrimps, the claw (or chela) of one of the first pair of walking legs is greatly enlarged. This claw can be closed rapidly to produce an audible snap. A snap produced against the body of a conspecific is capable of causing severe injury.

Not surprisingly, crustaceans often use these and similar weapons in aggressive displays; the weapons are extended, waved, or otherwise brandished during agonistic encounters. Such displays may function to signal aggressive intentions; in particular, brandishing a weapon may signal that attack is imminent. A weapon display also may serve to signal fighting ability, if weapon size is important in defeating opponents, or if weapon size correlates with body size and body size is important in defeating opponents.

The idea that weapons function to signal fighting ability has also been suggested for other categories of weapons, such as antlers of deer and the horns of sheep, however, the empirical evidence for a signal function of weapons is slim in all these groups. **We believe that the evidence is stronger for crustaceans, which is one reason for concentrating on these animals; the other is that weapon displays in crustaceans provide some of the best evidence of deception available for any type of aggressive signal.**

첫 단락에서 저자는 무기로 사용되는 갑각류의 부속기관(crustacean appendages)의 몇 가지 예를 설명하고 있다. 두 번째 단락은 그런 무기들이 디스플레이용으로도 사용된다는 사실을 말해준다. 세 번째 단락의 마지막에 가서야 다른 종류의 무기를 가진 동물이 아닌 갑각류를 연구의 주제로 선택한 이유가 등장한다: there is stronger evidence that crustacean weapons are used as signals of fighting ability, and they afford a unique opportunity to study deception.

| 문제점에서 해결책으로

단락을 배열하는 또 한 가지 방법은 글의 앞부분에서 문제 또는 패러독스를 제시한 뒤에 글을 진행하면서 문제를 해결하거나 문제를 해결할 수 있는 새로운 접근방식을 보여주는 것이다. 과학자는 끊임없이 앞선 연구결과를 재평가하고 논박하기 때문에 이런 유형의 배열이 흔하게 사용된다. 아래에 좋은 예가 있다.

When applied to ciliary propulsion, Lighthill's efficiency has some drawbacks. For one, it is not a direct criterion for the hydrodynamic efficiency of cilia as it also depends on the size and shape of the whole swimmer. Besides that, it is naturally applicable only for swimmers and not for other systems involving ciliary fluid transport with a variety of functions, like left-right asymmetry determination. **We therefore propose a different criterion for efficiency at the level of a single cilium or a carpet of cilia.** A first thought might be to define it as the volume flow rate of the transported fluid, divided by the dissipated power. However, as the flow rate scales linearly with the velocity, but the dissipation quadratically, this criterion would yield the highest efficiency for infinitesimally slow cilia, just like optimizing the fuel consumption of a road vehicle alone might lead to fitting it with an infinitesimally weak engine. Instead, like engineers trying to optimize the fuel consumption at a given speed, the well-posed question is which beating pattern of a cilium will achieve a certain flow rate with the smallest possible dissipation **The problem of finding the optimal strokes of hypothetical microswimmers has drawn a lot of attention in recent years.** Problems that have been solved include the optimal stroke pattern of Purcell's. three-link swimmer, an ideal elastic flagellum, a shape-changing body, a two-and a three-sphere swimmer, and a spherical squirmer. Most recently, Tam and Hosoi optimized the stroke patterns of *Chlamydomonas flagella.* **However, all these studies are still far from the complexity of a ciliary beat with an arbitrary 3D shape, let alone from an infinite field of interacting cilia. In addition, they were all performed for the swimming efficiency of the whole microorganism, whereas our goal is to optimize the pumping efficiency at the level of a single cilium,** which can be applicable to a much greater variety of ciliary systems.

저자는 일련의 문제점과 해결책을 제시하고 있다. 첫 단락에 묘사된 문제점에는 ciliary propulsion 효율에 관한 어느 계산법의 한계가 포함된다. 두 번째 단락에서 제기된 다른 문제점에는 하나의 미생물 개체에 기초한 계산의 초점이 너무 협소하다는 사실이 포함된다. 두 번째 단락의 끝부분에서 저자는 이러한 문제점들을 해결할 수 있는 개념적인 해결책, 즉 개별 cilium(cilia의 단수형)의 효율을 이해하는 방법을 제안한다.

| 비교와 대조

비교 또는 대조하는 패턴의 배열에서는 저자가 보통 한 단락에서는 어떤 주인공 또는 아이디어의 속성을 설명하고 다른 단락에서는 이와 비슷하거나 상이한 주인공 또는 아이디어를 설명하게 된다. 이런 순서를 사용하면 독자는 주인공을 분리해서 이들의 유사성 또는 차이점을 평가할 수 있다. 하나의 주인공 또는 아이디어를 설명하는 여러 개의 단락은 한 묶음으로 묶거나 아니면 단락마다 서로 다른 주인공이 번갈아 등장할 수도 있다. 딱정벌레에 관한 논문의 결과 섹션에서 발췌한 좋은 예를 살펴보자.

Males of *O. acuminatus* employed two very different tactics to encounter and mate with females: they either attempted to monopolize access to a female by **guarding** the entrance to her tunnel (guarding), or they attempted to bypass guarding males (**sneaking**). **Guarding** behavior entailed remaining inside a tunnel with a female, and fighting intruding males over possession of the tunnel. Guarding males blocked tunnel entrances and periodically "patrolled" the length of the tunnel. Rival males could gain possession of a tunnel only by forcibly evicting the resident male, and both fights and turnovers were frequent. Fights over tunnel occupancy entailed repeated butting, wrestling and pushing of opponents, and fights continued until one of the contestants left the tunnel.

Sneaking involved bypassing the guarding male. The primary method of sneaking into tunnels was to dig side-tunnels that intercepted guarded tunnels below ground. New tunnels were dug immediately adjacent (< 2 cm) to a guarded tunnel. These tunnels then turned horizontally 1-2 cm below ground, and often intercepted primary tunnels beneath the guarding male (16/24 side-tunnels). In this fashion, sneaking males sometimes bypassed the guarding male and mated with females undetected (observed in four instances).

저자는 첫 번째 단락에서 guarding과 sneaking을 소개한다. 그리고, 첫 단락의 나머지는 guarding을 설명하고 그 다음에 sneaking을 설명하는 데 할애된다. 이런 방식의 배열은 독자가 이 두 행태간의 차이를 쉽게 구별할 수 있게 도와준다.

모든 단락이 지금 설명된 패턴대로 배열되어 있는 것은 아니다. 다수의 단락이 앞 단락의 주제를 단순히 추가적으로 설명하거나 하나의 결과를 뒷받침하는 비슷한 무게의 증거를 제공하곤 한다. 과학저널의 한 논문에서 발췌한 아래의 서론을 살펴보자.

Bacteria form intimate and quite often mutually beneficial associations with a variety of multicellular organisms. The diversity of these associations, combined with their agricultural and clinical importance have made them a prominent focus of research. Of microbial genomes completed or under way, more than two- thirds are organisms that are either pathogens of humans or dependent on a close interaction with a eukaryotic host. But current databases and scientific literature present a distorted view of bacterial diversity. Estimates of bacterial diversity from various environmental sources, including the biota from animal surfaces and digestive tracts, show **that pathogens represent a very small portion of the microbial species**. Potential hosts, especially humans with their broad geographic distribution and high population densities, are constantly besieged by bacteria in the environment, but most do not cause infection.

Not only are pathogenesis and symbiosis relatively rare among bacteria species, they are derived conditions within bacteria as a whole, as evident from the fact that bacteria existed well before their eukaryotic hosts. The appearance of the major groups of eukaryotes, whose diversification could proceed only after the origin of mitochondria by endosymbiosis, marks the initial availability of abundant suitable hosts. The mitochondria themselves derive from a single lineage within the alpha subdivision of the Proteobacteria; that is to say, they are nested near the tips of the overall bacterial phylogeny. Thus, the distribution of pathogens and symbionts in numerous divergent clades of bacteria reflects the repeated and independent acquisition of this life-style.

두 번째 단락에서 저자는 첫 번째 단락에서 소개된 사실(pathogenesis and symbioses are rare among bacteria)에 추가적인 내용을 덧붙인다(these associations evolved after the rise of eukaryotes and were derived repeatedly and independently through time).

| 연결어구의 재발견

6장에서 논의된 연결어구는 독자가 문장에서 문장으로, 단락에서 단락으로 쉽게 이동할 수 있도록 도와준다. 연결어구는 문장이나 단락 배열의 패턴이 시간적 순서인지 비교나 대조인지 예견해준다. 적절한 연결어구를 올바른 위치에 사용하면(보통 문장이나 단락의 시작) 독자가 앞으로 읽게 될 내용에 대해 더 잘 준비된다. 다음의 연결어구와 이들이 예견하는 배열 패턴을 살펴보자.

시간적 순서를 예견하는 연결어구:
first, second, third, initially, then, finally, in conclusion, thus, to conclude, to summarize, another, after, afterward, at last, before, presently, during, earlier, immediately, later, meanwhile, now, recently, simultaneously, subsequently.

일반적인 내용에서 구체적인 내용으로 진행될 것을 예견하는 연결어구:
for example, for instance, namely, specifically, to illustrate, accordingly, consequently, hence, so, therefore, thus.

가장 덜 중요한 내용에서 가장 중요한 내용으로 진행될 것을 예견하는 연결어구:
clearly, most importantly, the most serious, the most weighty, the foremost.

문제점에서 해결책으로 진행될 것을 예견하는 연결어구:
but, however, in spite of, nevertheless, nonetheless, notwithstanding, instead, still, yet.

비교나 대조로 진행될 것을 예견하는 연결어구:

similarly, also, in the same way, just as, so too, likewise, in comparison, however, in contrast, on the contrary, unlike, however, on the one hand... on the other hand.

연습문제

⑮ 연습문제의 글에서 저자는 단락 배열에 어떤 패턴을 사용하고 있는가? 이런 패턴을 예견하게 해주는 단어는 무엇인가? 부록2의 연습문제 해답에서 여러분의 답이 맞는지 확인해보라.

1. Previous studies have shown that animals produce different antipredator vocalizations for aerial and terrestrial predators. Most of these studies, however, have presented these two types of predators in different ways, potentially confounding the interpretation that prey distinguish between types of predators and not their location or behavior. Our results show that chickadees do not vocally discriminate between raptors and mammals when they are presented in similar ways, and thus the "chick-a-dee" call does not refer specifically to the type of predator. Instead, these vocal signals likely contain information about the degree of threat that a predator represents. Maneuverability (e.g., as measured by turning radius, or radial acceleration) is extremely important in determining the outcome of predator-prey interactions and is inversely related to wingspan and body size in birds. Body size may be a good predictor of risk for chickadees: Small raptors tend to be much more maneuverable than larger raptors and likely pose a greater threat.

2. We tend to take for granted the ability of our immune systems to free our bodies of infection and prevent its recurrence. In some people, however, parts of the immune system fail. In the most severe of these immunodeficiency diseases, adaptive immunity is completely absent, and death occurs in infancy from overwhelming infection unless heroic

measures are taken. Other less catastrophic failures lead to recurrent infections with particular types of pathogen, depending on the particular deficiency. Much has been learned about the functions of the different components of the human immune system through the study of these immunodeficiencies, many of which are caused by inherited genetic defects. More than 25 years ago, a devastating form of immunodeficiency appeared, the acquired immune deficiency syndrome, or AIDS, which is caused by an infectious agent, the human immunodeficiency viruses HIV-1 and HIV-2. This disease destroys T cells, dendritic cells, and macrophages bearing CD4, leading to infections caused by intracellular bacteria and other pathogens normally controlled by such cells. These infections are the major cause of death from this increasingly prevalent immunodeficiency disease.

부록 **1**

글쓰기를 위한 기초 문법

명료한 글쓰기를 위해 복잡한 문법용어를 잔뜩 알아야 하는 것은 아니다. 글쓰기를 위한 기초 문법만 알면 된다: 즉, 품사와 기본문장구조. 이 두 개념은 아래에 예와 함께 설명되어 있다.

| 품사

품사는 문장에서 각 단어가 수행하는 역할을 설명해준다.

❶ **명사**는 사람이나 장소, 사물, 아이디어의 이름을 가리키며 문장에서 주어나 목적어로 기능한다. 이 책에서는 두 종류의 명사에 초점이 맞춰졌다: 구상명사, 즉 vertebrates, genes, DNA와 같이 실존하는 사물을 가리키는 명사와 추상명사, 즉 understanding, interpretation, prediction과 같이 실존하지 않는 아이디어나 감정, 질을 가리키는 명사. 명사 앞에는 관사가 오는 경우가 많다: a, an, the.

Scientists have studied *the* **arms** of spiral **galaxies.**

이 문장에 등장하는 명사는 모두 구체적이다: scientists, arms, galaxies. Arms 앞에는 관사인 the가 있다.

❷ **대명사**는 명사를 대신한다. 흔히 사용되는 대명사는 다음과 같다: I, you, we, it,

they, this, that, those, who, which, what.

They have studied **them** to determine the origin of spiral structure.

대명사 they는 앞 예문의 scientists를 대신하며, 대명사 them은 arms를 대신한
다.

❸ **형용사**는 명사나 대명사를 설명하거나 수식한다.

Many scientists have studied the **beautiful** arms of **spiral** galaxies.

형용사 many는 scientists를, beautiful은 arms를, spiral은 galaxies를 수식한다.

❹ **동사**는 액션이나 상태를 보여준다.

Many scientists **have studied** the beautiful arms of spiral galaxies.

동사인 have studied는 취해진 액션을 설명한다.

❺ **동사 파생형**은 동사처럼 보이지만 형용사나 부사, 명사로서 기능한다.

The beautiful arms of spiral galaxies, **outlined** by luminous young stars,
have been the focus of many studies.

이 문장에서 have been은 동사다. Outlined는 동사인 outline의 파생형이며 명
사인 arms를 수식하는 형용사로서 기능한다.

❻ **부사**는 동사나 형용사, 다른 부사 또는 문장 전체를 수식한다. 부사는 when,
how, where, how often, to what exent와 같은 질문에 대답함으로써 해당 품사를
제한하거나 정의한다.

We can identify the link between density wave acceleration of molecular clouds and the subsequent birth of stars **most easily** and **unambiguously** in galaxies external to our own.

부사인 easily와 unambiguously는 동사인 can identify를 수식한다. 다른 부사인 most는 부사인 easily를 수식한다.

❼ 대부분의 **전치사**는 시공간에서의 위치를 보여준다. 예를 들면 다음과 같다: in, under, above, below, at, after, before, until, for, with, by. 하지만, as if, as, like와 같이 흔히 사용되는 소수의 전치사는 그렇지 않다.

Molecular clouds spend a large fraction **of** their time **within** the arms **of** spiral galaxies.

❽ **접속사**는 문장의 구성요소 또는 문장과 문장 사이를 연결한다. 흔히 사용되는 접속사는 다음과 같다: and, but, or, nor, for, yet, so, however, consequently, therefore, because.

Many scientists have studied the beautiful arms of spiral galaxies outlined by luminous young stars, **but** the origin of spiral structure **and** the trigger for star formation remains unclear.

| 문장구조

문장구조란 단어나 구, 절을 가지고 문장이 만들어지는 방식을 가리킨다.

❶ 문장에서 주된 액션을 나타내는 단어는 **동사**이며 문장구조를 파악하는 좋은 시작점은 바로 동사를 찾는 것이다.

Many shorebirds <u>deplete</u> the prey.

이 문장의 동사는 deplete이며 이 단어는 액션을 설명해준다.

❷ **주어**는 문장이 말하고자 하는 대상이다. 동사 앞에서 "누가" 또는 "무엇이"라는 질문을 던지면 대개 주어를 찾을 수 있다.

Many <u>shorebirds</u> <u>deplete</u> the prey.

동사는 deplete이다. 누가 또는 무엇이 deplete이라는 액션을 수행하고 있는가. 답은 shorebirds이며 이 단어가 주어다.

❸ **목적어**란 동사의 액션을 받는 대상이다. 문장에는 목적어가 있을 수도, 없을 수도 있다. 대부분의 경우 동사 뒤에서 "누구를" 또는 "무엇을"이라는 질문을 던지면 목적어를 찾을 수 있다(아래 예문의 동그라미로 표시된).

Many <u>shorebirds</u> <u>deplete</u> the (prey.)

많은 shorebirds가 무엇을 deplete하는가? 대답은 바로 목적어인 prey다. 아래 예문에는 목적어가 없다.

The <u>shorebirds</u> <u>flew</u>.

❹ **절**이란 주어와 동사가 포함된 일군의 단어를 말한다. 절에는 독립절과 종속절이 있다. 두 개 또는 그 이상의 절이 하나의 문장을 구성하는 경우도 많다. 독립절은 주어와 동사를 모두 갖고 있으며 완결된 진술을 제공하기 때문에 홀로서기가 가능하다. 가장 단순한 문장이 바로 독립절이 된다.

When shorebirds deplete the prey in a small area, **the flock must move to a fresh site.**

이 문장의 독립절은 홀로서기가 가능한 부분이다: the flock must move to a fresh site. 이 독립절은 동사인 must move와 주어인 flock을 포함하며 완결된 진술을 제공한다.

종속절은 주어와 동사를 모두 갖고 있지만 홀로서기를 할 수 없다. 종속절은 완결된 진술을 하기 위해 독립절에 종속된다.

When shorebirds deplete the prey in a small area, the flock must move to a fresh site.

이 문장의 종속절은 다음과 같다: When shorebirds deplete the prey in a small area.

이 절은 종속어인 when으로 시작하기 때문에 진술을 완결할 수 없으며 동사인 deplete와 주어인 shorebirds가 있음에도 불구하고 홀로서기가 불가능하다.

다음에는 종속절을 시작할 때 흔히 사용되는 단어가 요약되어 있다.

after	since	whereas
although	so that	wherever
as	than	whether
because	though	whichever
as if	that	which
before	unless	while
even if	until	who
even though	what	whom
ever since	whatever	whose
how	when	why
if	whenever	where

❺ **구**란 주어와 동사가 없는 일군의 연관된 단어를 말한다. 구는 문장 내에서 주어, 수식어, 목적어로 기능할 수 있다. 이 책에서는 두 종류의 구에 초점이 맞추어졌다.

동사구는 동사파생어 및 이와 관련된 단어로 구성되며 다음 문장에서 괄호로 표시되어 있다.

Many shorebirds (feeding in a small area) <u>deplete</u> the prey.

동사구인 "feeding in a small area"는 shorebirds를 설명하는 형용사로 기능한다. Feeding은 동사파생어이며 그 뒤에 전치사구인 in a small area가 뒤따른다. 전치사구는 전치사와 목적어, 수식어로 구성되면 다음 문장에서 괄호로 표시되어 있다.

Many shorebirds (in a small area) <u>deplete</u> the prey.

전치사구인 in a small area는 shorebirds의 위치를 설명해준다. In은 전치사, area는 전치사의 목적어이며 small은 area를 수식해준다.

REFERENCE

1. Wilson, P. & Glazier, T. F. *The Least You Should Know about English* 8th edn (Wadsworth, 2003).

부록2
연습문제 해답

부록2에 제시된 교정문은 연습문제에 대한 유일한 해답이 아니다. 여러분이 더 좋은 해결책을 생각해낼 수도 있다. 이 교정문들을 길잡이로 활용해서 연습문제를 여러 번 다시 풀어보라. 연습을 통해서만 성장할 수 있다.

연습문제 ❶

1. <u>Processes</u> undertaken by diverse plants and animals <u>are</u> responsible for such ecological actions as nutrient cycling, carbon storage, and atmospheric regulation.

주어인 Processes가 추상적이다.

〈교정문〉

Diverse <u>plants</u> and <u>animals</u> <u>cycle</u> nutrients, <u>store</u> carbon, and <u>regulate</u> the atmosphere.

2. <u>Declines</u> in birth rates <u>have been observed</u> in many developed countries, and demographers expect that the transition to a stable population will eventually occur in many undeveloped nations as well.

주어인 Declines가 추상적이다.

<교정문>

Demographers <u>have observed</u> declines in birth rates in many developed countries and <u>expect</u> that eventually such declines will also lead to stable populations in many undeveloped nations.

3. <u>Variations</u> in magmatism during rifting <u>have been attributed</u> to variations in mantle temperature, rifting velocity or duration, active upwelling, or small-scale convection.

주어인 Variations가 추상적이다.

<교정문>

<u>Magmatism</u> <u>varies</u> during rifting for several reasons: changes in mantle temperature, rifting velocity or duration, active upwelling, or small-scale convection.

4. The <u>inability</u> of lateral variations in mantle temperature and composition, alone, to account for our observations <u>leads</u> us to propose that another influence was melt focusing.

주어인 Inability가 추상적이다.

<교정문>

<u>We</u> <u>could</u> not <u>account</u> for our observations with lateral variations in mantle temperature and composition alone. Another <u>influence</u> <u>was</u> melt focusing.

5. The <u>ability</u> of mudrock seals to prevent CO_2 leakage <u>is</u> a major concern for geological storage of anthropogenic CO_2.

주어인 ability가 추상적이다.

<교정문>

<u>Geologists</u> <u>are concerned</u> that mudrock seals may allow anthropogenic CO_2 to leak from geological storage.

연습문제 ❷

1. Photographs from space taken by satellites <u>are</u> indicators of urbanization and just one of the demonstrations of the human footprint.

<교정문>

Satellite photographs <u>indicate</u> the spread of urban areas and <u>demonstrate</u> the human footprint.

2. Weather variables (precipitation, temperature, and wind speed) <u>are</u> key factors in limiting summer habitat availability.

<교정문>

Precipitation, temperature, and wind speed <u>limit</u> available summer habitat.

3. A risk management ranking system <u>is</u> the central mechanism for which prioritization of terrestrial invasive species is based.

<교정문>

We <u>rank</u> terrestrial invasive species according to the threat they pose to the environment.

4. It <u>is</u> clear that Prairie Chickens are closely associated with sagebrush habitat throughout the year.

<교정문>

Prairie Chickens <u>occupy</u> sagebrush habitat throughout the year.

5. The occurrence of freezing and thawing <u>is</u> an important control on cohesive bank erosion in the region.

<교정문>

Freezing and thawing <u>control</u> cohesive bank erosion in the region.

연습문제 ❸

1. Environmentally sensitive <u>solutions</u> to the problems associated with continued population growth and development <u>will require</u> an environmentally literate citizenry.

<교정문>

To develop sustainable solutions to the problems of human growth and development, <u>we</u> <u>will need</u> environmentally literate citizens.

2. Partnerships between professional teachers, scientists, nonprofessional science educators, and administrators are needed to improve the content and effectiveness of science education, particularly in rural areas.

〈교정문〉

If we build partnerships between professional teachers, scientists, non-professional science educators, and administrators, we can improve the content and effectiveness of science education, particularly in rural areas.

3. Our ability to predict the spatial spread of exotic species and their transformation of natural communities is still developing.

〈교정문〉

We still cannot predict with certainty how an exotic species will spread or transform a natural community.

4. The amount of magmatism that accompanies the extension and rupture of the continental lithosphere varies dramatically at rifts and margins around the world.

〈교정문〉

When the continental lithosphere extends and ruptures at rifts and margins, the amount of accompanying magmatism varies dramatically.

5. The migration of melts vertically to the top of the melting region and then laterally along the base of the extended continental lithosphere would focus melts toward the eastern part of the basin.

<교정문>

Melts migrate vertically to the top of the melting region, then laterally along the base of the extended continental lithosphere toward the eastern part of the basin.

6. Pre-treatment of tenocytes with different concentrations of wortmannin (1, 10, and 20 nM) for 1h, treated with curcumin (5 μM) for 4 h, and then treated with IL-1β for 1h, inhibited the IL-1β-induced NF-κB activation.

<교정문>

The IL-1β-induced NF-κB activation was inhibited by pretreating tenocytes with wortmannin (1, 10, and 20 nM) for 1h, followed by curcumin (5μM) for 4h, and then IL-1β for 1h.

연습문제 ❹

1. Four big brown bats served as subjects in these experiments, two males and two females.

주어인 bats가 serving의 주체이기 때문에 동사인 served는 능동태이다.

2. The animals were collected from private homes in Maryland and were housed in the University of Maryland bat vivarium.

주어인 animals가 collecting 및 housing을 받는 대상이기 때문에 동사인 were collected와 were housed는 수동태이다.

3. Bats were maintained at 80% of their *ad lib* feeding weight and were normally fed mealworms only during experiments.

주어인 Bats가 maintain 및 feeding을 받는 대상이기 때문에 동사인 were maintained와 were fed는 수동태이다.

4. We <u>exposed</u> the bats to a reversed 12h dark:12h light cycle, and we gave them free access to water.

주어인 We가 exposing을 수행하고 있으며 따라서 동사인 exposed는 능동태이다.

연습문제 ⑤

1. For effective storage of industrial CO_2, retention times of ~10^4 yr or greater are required. (15 words)

<교정문>

Effective storage of industrial CO_2 requires retention times of ~10^4 yr or greater. (13 words)

2. It is hypothesized that groundwater pH must have been, on average, highest shortly before the Late Ordovician to Silurian proliferation of root-forming land plants. (24 words)

<교정문>

We hypothesized that, on average, groundwater pH must have been highest shortly before the Late Ordovician to Silurian proliferation of root-forming land plants. (23 words)

3. We were compelled to rely on the SOC90 data as no further information on the occupational situation (employed vs. selfemployed) or on the size of the firm was available in retrospective form. (32 words)

<교정문>

We relied on the SOC90 data because we couldn't find past information on the number of people who were employed versus self-employed or on the size of the firm. (29 words)

4. Moreover, it has been demonstrated that mineral-water reactions increase the pH of groundwater even in the presence of abundant acid-producing lichens (Schatz 1963). (24 words)

<교정문>

Schatz (1963) demonstrated that mineral-water reactions increase the pH of groundwater, even in the presence of abundant acid-producing lichens. (19 words)

연습문제 ⑥

1. For example, <u>expansion</u> of the extent of the winter range by <u>continued</u> <u>pioneering</u> of segments of the northern Yellowstone elk herd northward from the park <u>boundary</u> and <u>extensive</u> use of these more northerly areas by greater numbers of elk have been <u>coincident</u> with <u>acquisition</u> and <u>conversion</u> of rangelands from livestock <u>production</u> to elk winter range.

긴 단어

expansion: 3음절, 라틴어; continued: 3음절, 라틴어에서 유래한 오래된 불어; pioneering: 4음절, 오래된 불어; boundary: 3음절, 라틴어에서 유래한 오래된 불어; extensive: 3음절, 불어 또는 라틴어; coincident: 4음절, 라틴어; acquisition: 4음절, 라틴어; conversion: 3음절, 라틴어에서 유래한 오래된 불어; production: 3음절, 라틴어에서 유래한 오래된 불어.

For example, as ranchland north of the park boundary was <u>bought</u> and <u>put</u> into winter range, elk from the northern Yellowstone herd <u>shifted</u> north to <u>fill</u> it.

짧은 단어

bought: 1음절, 오래된 영어; put: 1음절, 오래된 영어; shift: 1음절, 오래된 영어; fill: 1음절, 오래된 영어.

2. We conclude that snag <u>retention</u> at <u>multiple</u> <u>spatial</u> and <u>temporal</u> scales in recent burns, which will be salvage-logged, is a <u>prescription</u> that must be <u>implemented</u> to meet the <u>principles</u> of <u>sustainable</u> forest <u>management</u> and the <u>maintenance</u> of biodiversity in the boreal forest.

긴 단어

retention: 3음절, 오래된 불어 또는 라틴어; multiple: 3음절, 라틴어; spatial: 2음절, 라틴어; temporal: 3음절, 오래된 불어 또는 라틴어; prescription: 3음절, 라틴어에서 유래한 오래된 불어; implemented: 4음절, 라틴어; principles: 3음절, 라티어; sustainable: 4음절, 라틴어; management: 3음절, 라틴어; maintenance: 3음절, 오래된 불어.

〈교정문〉

We <u>found</u> that leaving snags in salvage-logged burns <u>helped</u> <u>keep</u> biodiversity <u>high</u>.

짧은 단어

find: 1음절, 오래된 영어; leave: 1음절, 오래된 영어; help: 1음절, 오래된 영어; keep: 1음절, 오래된 영어; high: 1음절, 오래된 영어.

연습문제 ⑦

1. One way to assess the perceived risk of feeding in different <u>locations</u> is to measure the proportion of the available food a forager removes before switching to an alternative <u>patch</u>. All else being equal, foragers should be willing to forage longer and remove more food from a safe <u>area</u> than a risky one.

<교정문>

We can assess the perceived risk of feeding in different <u>patches</u> by measuring the proportion of the available food a forager removes before switching to an alternative <u>patch</u>. All else being equal, foragers should be willing to forage longer and remove more food from a safe <u>patch</u> than a risky one.

2. <u>Stress coping styles</u> have been characterized as a proactive/reactive dichotomy in laboratory and domesticated animals. In this study, we examined the prevalence of <u>proactive/reactive stress coping styles</u> in wild-caught short-tailed mice (*Scotinomys teguina*). We compared <u>stress responses</u> to spontaneous singing, a social and reproductive behavior that characterizes this species.

<교정문>

Studies show that many animals manage <u>stress</u> either proactively or reactively. Here we examine whether individual wildcaught short-tailed mice (*Scotinomys teguina*) are proactive or reactive in the way they manage <u>stress</u> in response to spontaneous singing — a characteristic social and reproductive behavior of the species.

3. <u>Antimicrobial resistance genes</u> allow a microorganism to expand its

ecological niche, allowing its proliferation in the presence of certain noxious compounds. From this standpoint, it is not surprising that antibiotic resistance genes are associated with highly mobile genetic elements, because the benefit to a microorganism derived from antibiotic resistance is transient, owing to the temporal and spatial heterogeneity of antibiotic-bearing environments.

〈교정문〉

Microbes can live and even proliferate in noxious environments thanks to antibiotic resistance genes. Antibiotic resistance genes are associated with highly mobile genetic elements that help microbes deal with constantly changing antibiotic-containing environments.

4. Studies of long-term outcomes in offspring exposed to maternal undernutrition and stress caused by the Dutch Hunger Winter of 1944 to 1945 revealed an increased prevalence of metabolic disease, such as glucose intolerance, obesity, and cardiovascular disease, as well as emotional and psychiatric disorders. Animal models have been developed to assess the long-term consequences of a variety of maternal challenges including under-and over-nutrition, hyperglycemia, chronic stress, and inflammation. Exposures to a wide range of insults during gestation are associated with convergent effects on fetal growth, neurodevelopment, and metabolism.

〈교정문〉

Studies show that when mothers starved during pregnancy in the Dutch Hunger Winter of 1944 to 1945, their children often developed metabolic diseases later in life, which included glucose intolerance, obesity, and cardiovascular disease as well as emotional and psychiatric disorders. Research on animals shows similar results: <u>starvation</u>, overeating, chronic stress, and inflammation during pregnancy influence fetal growth, neurodevelopment, and metabolism.

연습문제 ❽

1. Developing <u>regular exercise programs</u> and <u>diet regimes</u> contributes to <u>disease risk prevention</u> and <u>optimal health promotion</u>.

<교정문>

Regular exercise and attention to diet help prevent disease and promote health.

2. Research focused on <u>care time deficits</u> and <u>time squeezes</u> for families has identified the persistence of <u>gendered care time burdens</u> and the sense of <u>time pressure</u> many <u>dual-earner families</u> experience around care.

<교정문>

Research on families where both parents work shows that the demands of child care are stressful and still met largely by mothers.

3. There will be <u>major conservation implications</u> if <u>mercury ingestion</u> in ospreys causes <u>negative population level effects</u> either through <u>direct mortality</u> or <u>negative fecundity</u>.

<교정문>

If ospreys decline because ingesting mercury either kills them directly or lowers their breeding success, we face a serious conservation problem.

연습문제 ⑨

1. One of the well-researched immunoregulatory functions of probiotics is the induction of cytokine production. In particular, the induction of IL-10 and IL-12 production by probiotics has been studied intensively, because the balance of IL-10 / IL-12 secreted by macrophages and dendritic cells in response to microbes is crucial for determination of the direction of the immune response. IL-10 is an anti-inflammatory cytokine and is expected to improve chronic inflammation, such as that of inflammatory bowel disease and autoimmune disease. IL-10 downregulates phagocytic and T cell functions, including the production of proinflammatory cytokines, such as IL-12, TNF-α, and IFN-γ, that control inflammatory responses. IL-10 promotes the development of regulatory T cells for the control of excessive immune responses. In contrast, IL-12 is an important mediator of cell-mediated immunity and is expected to augment the natural immune defense against infections and cancers. IL-12 stimulates T cells to secrete IFN-γ, promotes Th1 cell development, and, directly or indirectly, augments the cytotoxic activity of NK cells and macrophages. IL-12 also suppresses redundant Th2 cell responses for the control of allergy.

저자는 독자에게 익숙하지 않을 수 있는 두 개의 테크니컬 용어를 소개하고 있다: IL-10(Interleukin-10), IL-12(Interleukin-12). 저자는 이 두 용어를 학부 수준의 면역학 지식이 있는 독자가 이해할 수 있도록 설명하고 있다. 저자는 독자에게 이 두 가지가 cytokine이라는 사실과 이들이 면역계에서 수행하는 역할에 관해 설명해준다. IL-10은 항염증작용을 하며 대식세포와 T세포의 기능을 억제하는 한 편 조절 T 세포(regulatory T cells)의 발달을 촉진시킨다. IL-12는 세포매개면역 반응에 관여하며 T 세포를 활성화시키고 불필요한 Th2 세포 반응을 억제한다.

연습문제 ⑩

1. While a growing body of research indicates that large herbivores as a group can exert strong indirect effects on co-occurring species, there are comparatively few examples of strong community-wide impacts from

individual large herbivore species. (37 words)

While a growing body of는 불필요한 디테일이다; indicates는 모호한 표현이다; as a group은 중복이다; can exert strong indirect effects는 더 짧게 표현될 수 있다; comparatively few는 모호한 표현이다; individual large herbivore species는 두 개의 명사 및 두 개의 형용사로 이루어진 문자열이다.

<교정문>

Research shows that large herbivores can indirectly influence co-occurring species, but few studies focus on a single species of large herbivore and how it affects the whole community. (28 words)

2. Small mammal species diversity increased in exclosures relative to controls, while survivorship showed no significant trends. (16 words)

Small mammal species diversity는 하나의 형용사 및 세 개의 명사로 구성된 문자열이다; species는 중복이다; no significant trends는 부정적 표현이다.

<교정문>

Diversity of small mammals increased in exclosures relative to controls, while survivorship stayed the same. (15 words)

3. In this essay, I will be looking at how higher summer temperatures cause quicker soil and plant evaporation. We all know that climate change has caused elevated temperatures in the Northwest throughout the spring and summer months. We also know that these record-breaking temperatures have the effect of quickly and easily desiccating soil and drying out plant foliage so that it is more flammable. Understandably then, when lightning strikes this very combustible environment, a spark

can very quickly turn into a widespread blaze. (83 words)

다음과 같은 표현은 모두 과도한 연결어구이다: In this essay I will be looking at how, We all know that, We also know that these, Understandably then; higher summer temperatures와 record-breaking temperatures는 반복되는 표현이며 더 짧게 표현될 수 있다; more flammable과 very combustible environment는 반복이다; widespread blaze는 더 짧게 표현될 수 있다.

<교정문>

Due to climate change, spring and summer temperatures in the Northwest are becoming warmer. Warmer temperatures dry out both soils and plant foliage, which are then more prone to wildfires. (30 words)

4. Zimbabwean undocumented migrants are shown to be marginalized and vulnerable with limited transnational citizenship. (14 words)

Zimbabwean undocumented migrants는 두 개의 형용사와 하나의 명사로 이루어진 거추장스럽게 긴 문자열이다; are shown to be는 수동태 동사이며 알려지지 않은 관찰자가 있다는 사실을 나타낸다 – 이 것 역시 과도한 연결어구의 한 종류이다.

<교정문>

Undocumented migrants from Zimbabwe are marginalized and vulnerable with limited transnational citizenship. (12 words)

5. When the lithosphere extends and rifts along continental margins, magma is produced in varying quantities. Widely spaced geophysical transects show that rifting along some continental margins can transition from

magma-poor to magma-rich. Our wide-angle seismic data from the Black Sea provide the first direct observations of such a transition. This transition coincides with a transform fault and is abrupt, occurring over only ~20–30 km. This abrupt transition cannot be explained solely by gradual along-margin variations in mantle properties, since these would be expected to result in a smooth transition from magma-poor to magma-rich rifting over hundreds of kilometers. We suggest that the abruptness of the transition results from the 3-D migration of magma into areas of greater extension during rifting, a phenomenon that has been observed in active rift environments such as mid-ocean ridges. (133 words)

이 예문은 그 자체로 좋은 글이다.

6. The empirical data presented in this article reveal a segmented labor market and exploitation, with undocumented migrants not benefiting from international protection, human rights, nation state citizenship rights, or rights associated with the more recent concepts of post-national and transnational citizenship. (41 words)

The empirical data presented in this article은 과도한 연결어구이다.

<교정문>

The segmented labor market we describe exploits undocumented migrants. These people lack international protection, human rights, nation-state citizenship, and rights associated with the more recent concepts of postnational and transnational citizenship. (30 words)

7. The systemic immune response in *Drosophila* is mediated by a battery of antimicrobial peptides produced largely by the fat body, an insect organ analogous to the mammalian liver. These peptides lyse microorganisms

by forming pores in their cell walls. Functionally, the antimicrobial peptides fall into three classes depending on the pathogen specificity of their lytic activity. Thus, Drosomycin is a major antifungal peptide, whereas Diptericin is active against gram-negative bacteria, and Defensin works against gram-positive bacteria. Interestingly, infection of *Drosophila* with different classes of pathogens leads to preferential induction of the appropriate group of antimicrobial peptides.

사용된 연결어구는 다음과 같다: functionally, thus, whereas, interestingly. 이런 단어는 저자가 antimicrobial peptides의 역할을 설명하고, 목록의 아이템을 분명하게 드러내고, 흥미로운 사실을 지적할 때 독자가 저자의 생각의 흐름을 따라갈 수 있도록 도와준다.

8. Introgressive hybridization is most commonly observed in zones of geographical contact between otherwise allopatric taxa. Studies of such zones have provided important insights into the evolutionary process and have helped resolve part of the debate about fitness of hybrids. In many cases, most hybrid genotypes tend to be less fit than are the parental genotypes in parental habitats, owing either to endogenous or exogenous selection or both. However, theory predicts that some can be of equal or superior fitness in new habitats and, occasionally, even in parental habitats.

이 예문에서는 쉬운 영어의 많은 원칙이 분명하게 드러난다: 주어 뒤에 동사가 뒤따른다; 하나를 제외하고는 능동태 동사가 사용되었으며, 수동태인 is most commonly observed도 저자가 Introgressive hybridization을 주어로 사용할 수 있게 해주는 역할을 한다; 불필요한 연결어구가 없고, 부정적 표현, 반복이나 과도한 세부사항도 있다. 한 마디로 간결하다.

연습문제 ⑪

1. Unfortunately, as noted 40 years ago, few students experience the

thrill of doing field science because they are rarely allowed to leave the confines of the classroom to become immersed in field-based science.

저자는 이 예문에서 오래된 정보를 문장의 마지막에 두고 있다: to become immersed in field-based science.

<교정문>

Unfortunately, as noted 40 years ago, few students experience the thrill of doing field science because they are rarely allowed to leave the confines of the classroom.

2. Bank erosion rates along the South River in Virginia increased by factors of 2–3 after 1957. Increased bank erosion rates cannot be explained by changes in the intensity of either freeze-thaw or storm intensity, and changes in the density of riparian trees should have decreased erosion rates.

이 두 문장의 주어는 일관적이다: bank erosion rates; 하지만 오래된 정보가 두 번째 문장의 마지막에 잘못 배치되어 있다: decreased erosion rates. 두 번째 문장에는 부정적 표현인 cannot be explained가 사용되었다.

<교정문>

After 1957, bank erosion in Southern Virginia increased by 2–3 times. These increases have little to do with the severity of freeze-thaw cycles, or with the intensity of storms, and changes in the density of riparian trees should have had a stabilizing effect.

3. Students majoring in science often believe they can escape the intensive writing and presentations that their peers in the humanities and social

sciences must do. However, science is a collective human endeavor whose success hinges upon effective communication, both written and oral. Even if findings are ground breaking, they are potentially worthless if they can't be shared with others in a clear and engaging way. Teaching undergraduate science students to effectively communicate is therefore an essential goal.

이 단락의 주어는, 수식어까지 포함한다면, 상당히 일관적이다: students (majoring in science), science, findings(이 경우 findings in science라는 점이 자명함), teaching(science students). 첫 세 문장은 새로운 정보를 숨기는 불필요한 단어들로 끝난다.

〈교정문〉

Science students often believe they can escape the intensive writing and presentations of their peers in the humanities and social sciences. However, science is a collective human endeavor whose success hinges upon effective communication. Even if findings are ground breaking, they are potentially worthless if they can't be shared; therefore, teaching undergraduate science students to communicate effectively is an essential goal.

4. Climate plays an important part in determining the average numbers of a species, and periodical seasons of extreme cold or drought, I believe to be the most effective of all checks. I estimated that the winter of 1854–55 destroyed four-fifths of the birds in my own grounds; and this is a tremendous destruction, when we remember that ten per cent is an extraordinarily severe mortality from epidemics with man. The action of climate seems at first sight to be quite independent of the struggle for existence; but in so far as climate chiefly acts in reducing food, it brings on the most severe struggle between the individuals, whether of the

same or of distinct species, which subsist on the same kind of food. Even when climate, for instance extreme cold, acts directly, it will be the least vigorous, or those which have got least food through the advancing winter, which will suffer most.

이 글은 찰스 다윈의 종의 기원에서 발췌한 것이다. 각 문장이 새로운 정보와 오래된 정보가 어떻게 배치되어야 하는지에 관한 좋은 예이다.

연습문제 ⑫

1. Central to this deficit has been the rising average age of the nursing workforce and the decline in the number of hours worked; fewer nurses are working standard full-time hours (35-44 hours per week) and 44 percent work part-time.

이 문장에는 두 개의 목록이 있으며 어느 것도 평행구조를 갖지 않는다. 첫 목록의 아이템은 다음과 같다:

the rising average age of the nursing workforce, and
the decline in the number of hours worked

교정하기 위해서는 nursing workforce는 nurses로, decline은 declining으로 바꾸라. 그러면 다음과 같이 된다:
the rising average age of nurses and
the declining number of hours worked

두 번째 목록의 아이템은 다음과 같다:

fewer nurses are working standard full-time hours (35-44 hours per week), and
44 percent work part-time

교정하기 위해서는 standard와 hours를 삭제하고 more nurses와 working을 추가하라. 44 percent는 문장 끝으로 옮기라. 그러면 다음과 같이 된다:

fewer nurses are working standard full-time (35-44 hours per week), and more nurses are working part-time (44 percent).

두 번째 등장하는 nurses도 생략이 가능하다.

<교정문>

Central to this deficit has been the rising average age of nurses and the declining number of hours worked; fewer nurses are working full- time (35–44 hours per week), and more are working part- time (44 percent).

2. The problem of finding the optimal strokes of hypothetical microswimmers has drawn a lot of attention in recent years. Problems that have been solved include the optimal stroke pattern of Purcell's three-link swimmer, an ideal elastic flagellum, a shape-changing body, a two- and a three-sphere swimmer, and a spherical squirmer.

목록을 소개하는 새로운 정보가 첫 문장의 앞에 등장한다: The problem of finding the optimal strokes of hypothetical microswimmers. 목록도 평행구조가 아니다:

the optimal stroke pattern of Purcell's three-link swimmer,
an ideal elastic flagellum,
a shape-changing body,
a two- and three-sphere swimmer, and
a spherical squirmer.

목록을 소개하는 정보를 문장의 끝에 두라: optimal strokes of hypothetical

microswimmers. 두 번째 문장에서 Optimal strokes를 주어로 사용하고 동일한 단어인 for를 이용해서 목록의 각 아이템을 소개하라 (첫 아이템 후부터는 for를 반복할 필요가 없다. 그러면 다음과 같이 된다:

for Purcell's three-link swimmer,
an ideal elastic flagellum,
a shape-changing body,
a two- and three-sphere swimmer, and
a spherical squirmer.

〈교정문〉

In recent years, much attention has focused on finding the optimal strokes of hypothetical microswimmers. Optimal strokes have been found for Purcell's three-link swimmer, an ideal elastic flagellum, a shape-changing body, a two- and three-sphere swimmer, and a spherical squirmer.

3. Cilia are hair-like protrusions that beat in an asymmetric fashion to pump the fluid in the direction of their effective stroke. They propel certain protozoa, such as *Paramecium*, and also fulfill a number of functions in mammals, including mucous clearance from airways, left-right asymmetry determination, and transport of an egg cell in fallopian tubes.

두 번째 문장의 새로운 정보는 문장의 앞과 중간에 등장한다(propel certain protozoa, fulfill a number of functions). Functions는 추상적이며 목록은 평행구조가 아니다:

mucous clearance in airways,
left-right asymmetry determination, and
transport of an egg cell in fallopian tubes.

짧은 문장으로 목록을 소개한 뒤 different organisms로 문장을 마치라. 각 종류의 organism을 한 문장으로 소개하고 문장을 유사한 단어로 시작하라: In protozoa, In mammals. 그리고 문장을 새로운 정보로 마무리하라. 각 아이템을 하나의 현재시제 동사로 소개함으로써 목록을 평행구조로 만들라:

clear mucous from airways,
determine left-right asymmetry, and
transport egg cells in fallopian tubes.

〈교정문〉

Cilia are hair-like protrusions that beat asymmetrically to pump fluid in the direction of their effective stroke. This pumping is put to an astonishing variety of uses by different organisms. In protozoa such as *Paramecium*, cilia provide the primary power for movement. In mammals, cilia clear mucous from airways, determine left-right asymmetry, and transport egg cells in fallopian tubes.

4. Integrons consist of three elements: an attachment site where the horizontally acquired sequence is integrated; a gene encoding a site-specific recombinase (that is, integrase); and a promoter that drives expression of the incorporated sequence.

목록이 평행구조가 아니다.

attachment site where the horizontally acquired sequence is integrated;
a gene encoding a site-specific recombinase (that is, integrase); and
a promoter that drives expression of the encorporated sequence.

각 아이템의 that으로 동일하게 시작하며 현재시제 동사가 사용되는 종속절을 붙이라. 그러면 다음과 같이 된다:

an attachment site that locates the integration of the horizontally acquired sequence;

a gene that encodes a site-specific recombinase (that is, integrase); and

a promoter that drives expression of the incorporated sequence.

<교정문>

Integrons consist of three elements: an attachment site that locates the integration of the horizontally acquired sequence; a gene that encodes a site-specific recombinase (that is, integrase); and a promoter that drives expression of the incorporated sequence.

5. North American (NA)-EEEV strains cause periodic outbreaks of mosquito-borne encephalitis in humans and equines, are highly neurovirulent, and, in comparison with related Venezuelan equine encephalitis virus (VEEV) and western equine encephalitis virus (WEEV), cause far more severe encephalitic disease in humans.

목록이 평행구조가 아니다. 세 아이템 각각은 현재시제 동사로 시작한다: cause, are, cause. 각 동사 뒤에는 목적어 및 목적어의 수식어가 따른다: periodic outbreaks, highly neurovirulent, far more severe encephalitic disease.

연습문제 ⑬

1. In order to unravel the mode of action of neuronal networks, a neurobiologist's dream would be not only to be able to monitor neuronal activity but also to have control over distinct sets of neurons and to be able to manipulate their activity and observe the effect on behavior. (49 words) This idea is not new. (5 words) As the activity of a neuron is based on the depolarization of its cell membrane, neuronal activity can be induced by an experimenter using stimulation electrodes by which the cell membrane can be artificially depolarized or hyperpolarized.

(37 words) Although stimulation electrodes have served, and continue to serve, neuroscientists well for decades, limitations of this invasive approach are obvious. (20 words)

이 예문에는 5단어에서 49단어에 이르는 다양한 길이의 문장이 등장한다. 문장 당 평균 단어수는 28로서 길다. 불필요한 단어를 제거함으로써 문장 길이를 줄일 수 있다. 예를 들어, 첫 문장인 아래 문장은:

In order to unravel the mode of action of neuronal networks, a neurobiologist's dream would be not only to be able to monitor neuronal activity but also to have control over distinct sets of neurons and to be able to manipulate their activity and observe the effect on behavior. (49 words)

다음과 같이 교정될 수 있다;

Neurobiologists dream of being able to monitor neuronal activity and control and manipulate distinct sets of neurons, while at the same time observing how these changes affect behavior. (28 words)

2. The extrapolation from *in vitro* measurements to the *in vivo* behavior of proteins is hampered by extremely high (300-400 mg/mL) intracellular macromolecular concentrations in the cell, i.e. crowding, which is one of the most important factors that influences the structure and function of proteins under physiological conditions. (47 words)

이 문장은 너무 길다. 쪼갠 뒤에 중요한 정보를 문장의 마지막에 두라.

<교정문>

One of the most important factors influencing the structure and function of proteins under physiological conditions is crowding. (18 words) Crowding occurs when extremely high (300–400 mg/mL) concentrations of intracellular macromolecules occur in the cell, making it hard to extrapolate from *in vitro* measurements to the proteins' *in vivo* behavior. (30 words)

3. Some of the confusion about the role of hybridization in evolutionary diversification stems from the contradiction between a perceived necessity for cessation of gene flow to enable adaptive population differentiation on the one hand, and the potential of hybridization for generating adaptive variation, functional novelty, and new species on the other. (52 words)

이 문장은 너무 길다. 쪼개서 각 문장이 하나 또는 최대 두 개의 주요 아이디어를 담도록 만들라.

<교정문>

Whether interspecific hybridization is important as a mechanism that generates biological diversity is controversial. (14 words) While some authors see hybrids as a source of genetic variation, functional novelty, and new species, others argue that reduced fitness would typically render hybrids an evolutionary dead end. (29 words)

연습문제 ⑭

1. Males of O. *acuminatus* [dung beetles] employed two very different tactics to encounter and mate with females: they either attempted to monopolize access to a female by guarding the entrance to her tunnel (guarding), or they attempted to bypass guarding males (sneaking).

Guarding behavior entailed remaining inside a tunnel with a female, and fighting intruding males over possession of the tunnel. Guarding males blocked tunnel entrances and periodically "patrolled" the length of the tunnel. Rival males could gain possession of a tunnel only by forcibly evicting the resident male, and both fights and turnovers were frequent. Fights over tunnel occupancy entailed repeated butting, wrestling and pushing of opponents, and fights continued until one of the contestants left the tunnel.

첫 문장이 이슈를 제기한다. 저자는 이 문장에서 dung beetles가 암컷을 만나고 교미하기 위해 사용하는 두 가지 전략을 소개한다: guarding과 sneaking. Guadrding 행태에 관한 설명이 발전에서 이어진다.

2. One prerequisite for the maintenance of dimorphism is that organisms experience a fitness tradeoff across environments. If animals encounter several discrete environment types, or ecological or behavioral situations, and these different environments favor different morphologies, then distinct morphological alternatives can evolve within a single population—each specialized for one of the different environments. Such fitness tradeoffs have been demonstrated for several dimorphic species. For example, soft and hard seed diets have favored two divergent bill morphologies within populations of African finches, and high and low levels of predation have favored alternative shell morphologies in barnacles, and spined and spineless morphologies in rotifers and *Daphnia*. It is possible that the alternative reproductive tactics characterized in this study produce a similar situation in *O. acuminatus*. If guarding and sneaking behaviors favor horned and hornless male morphologies, respectively, then the reproductive behavior of males may have contributed to the evolution of male horn length dimorphism in this species.

첫 세 문장이 이슈를 제기한다. 저자는 서로 다른 환경에서 일어나는 evolution 과 dimorphism의 유지에 관한 개념을 소개한다. 이슈의 마지막 문장은 발전에서 등장할 내용을 소개한다: a list of examples of several dimorphic species whose fitness tradeoffs have been demonstrated.

3. In recent times, the origin of the adaptive immune response has been uncovered. It turns out that the two recombinase-activated genes are encoded in a short stretch of DNA, in opposite orientations and lacking exons. This suggested an origin in a retroposon, as did the presence of the recognition signal sequences that lie 3' of all V gene segments and 5' of all J gene segments. This hypothesis was tested *in vitro* and shown to be true. Other processes expand diversity tremendously, such as the generation of D gene segments in the first chain to rearrange, the nucleotide-adding enzyme TdT that inserts nucleotides in the junctions of V-D-J junctions, and somatic hypermutation.

첫 문장이 이슈를 제기한다. 저자는 adaptive immune response의 기원에 관한 개념을 소개한 다음 발전 부분에서 유전적 기원의 상세내용으로 확장하고 있다.

4. Despite a consistent correlation between genome size and the obligate association with host cells, genome reduction is not simply an adaptive response to living within hosts. Instead, the trend toward large-scale gene loss reflects a lack of effective selection for maintaining genes in these specialized microbes. Because the host presents a constant environment rich in metabolic intermediates, some genes are rendered useless by adoption of a strictly symbiotic or pathogenic life-style. These superfluous sequences are eliminated through mutational bias favoring deletions, a process apparently universal in bacterial lineages. Thus, all of the fully sequenced small genomes display a pattern of loss of biosynthetic pathways, such as those for amino acids that can be obtained from the host cytoplasm.

첫 두 문장이 이슈를 제기한다. 저자는 하나의 전제를 세운 뒤에 이를 반박한다: Despite a constant correlation ⋯ genome reduction is not simply an adaptive response ⋯ and Instead ⋯ large scale genome loss ⋯ reflects a lack of ⋯ selection for maintaining genes ⋯ 발전에서는 selection이 일어나지 않은 이유가 설명되며 결론은 이를 요약해준다.

5. Unlike pathogens, symbionts may devote part of their genomes to processes that are more directly beneficial to the host rather than to the bacterial cell itself. *Buchnera* retains and even amplifies genes for the biosynthesis of amino acids required by hosts, devoting almost 10% of its genome to these pathways, which are missing from pathogens with similarly small genomes. Because of their fastidious growth requirements, the biological role of obligately associated symbionts can rarely be determined experimentally. However, genome comparisons can provide a means for determining their functions in hosts. Such future research should reveal, for example, whether the endosymbionts of blood-feeding hosts, such as *Wigglesworthia glossinia* in tsetse flies, retain pathways for biosynthesis of vitamins absent from blood, whether the symbiont *Vibrio fischeri* provides functions other than bioluminescence to its squid host, and whether the mutualistic *Wolbachia* of filarial nematodes contain genes for host benefit that are absent in the parasitic *Wolbachia* of arthropods.

첫 문장이 이슈를 제기한다. 저자는 이 문장에서 symbionts가 숙주(hosts)를 이롭게 하는 프로세스에 genome의 일부를 할애할 수 있다는 개념을 소개한다. 발전에서는 이런 종류의 symbiont의 예가 소개된다. 결론은 추측으로서 obligate symbionts에 관한 앞으로의 연구가 밝혀야 할 내용을 그리고 있다.

연습문제 ⓯

1. Previous studies have shown that animals produce different antipredator vocalizations for aerial and terrestrial predators. Most of these studies,

however, have presented these two types of predators in different ways, potentially confounding the interpretation that prey distinguish between types of predators and not their location or behavior. Our results show that chickadees do not vocally discriminate between raptors and mammals when they are presented in similar ways, and thus the "chick-a-dee" call does not refer specifically to the type of predator. Instead, these vocal signals likely contain information about the degree of threat that a predator represents. Maneuverability (e.g., as measured by turning radius, or radial acceleration) is extremely important in determining the outcome of predator-prey interactions and is inversely related to wingspan and body size in birds. Body size may be a good predictor of risk for chickadees: Small raptors tend to be much more maneuverable than larger raptors and likely pose a greater threat.

저자는 첫 단락에서 앞 연구의 문제점을 설명하고 있다. vocalization 실험에서 experiments에서 포식자(육상동물이건 공중동물이건 간에)를 피식자 동물에게 제시하는 방식이 결과에 혼동을 줄 수 있다. 저자는 두 번째 단락에서 이에 대한 해결책을 제시하며 포식자가 동일한 방식으로 제시될 경우 피식자는 포식자가 육상동물이나 공중동물이라는 사실보다 포식의 체구와 기술을 더 중요하게 여긴다는 점을 보여준다.

저자는 두 번째 단락을 instead로 시작하며 이 단어는 해당 단락이 문제점에 접근하는 새로운 방식을 제시하리라는 점을 미리 알려준다.

2. We tend to take for granted the ability of our immune systems to free our bodies of infection and prevent its recurrence. In some people, however, parts of the immune system fail. In the most severe of these immunodeficiency diseases, adaptive immunity is completely absent, and death occurs in infancy from overwhelming infection unless heroic measures are taken. Other less catastrophic failures lead to recurrent infections with particular types of pathogen, depending on the particular deficiency. Much has been learned about the functions of the different

components of the human immune system through the study of these immunodeficiencies, many of which are caused by inherited genetic defects.

More than 25 years ago, a devastating form of immunodeficiency appeared, the acquired immune deficiency syndrome, or AIDS, which is caused by an infectious agent, the human immunodeficiency viruses HIV-1 and HIV-2. This disease destroys T cells, dendritic cells, and macrophages bearing CD4, leading to infections caused by intracellular bacteria and other pathogens normally controlled by such cells. These infections are the major cause of death from this increasingly prevalent immunodeficiency disease.

저자는 이 두 단락에서 일반적인 정보에서 구체적인 정보로 진행하고 있다. 첫 단락은 immunodeficiency disease에 관한 짧은 리뷰이다. 두 번째 단락은 특정 종류의 immunodeficiency disease, 즉 AIDS에 초점을 맞춘다.

이런 배열에 관해 예견해주는 어떤 단어도 사용되지 않았지만 저자는 더 섬세한 기법을 이용해 이 두 단락을 연결하고 있다. 저자는 첫 문장을 시간과 관련한 간접적인 언급으로 마친다: Much has been learned about the functions of the different components of the human immune system through the study of these immunodeficiencies. 그런 다음 두 번째 단락을 첫 번째 단락의 시간과 공명하는, 시간과 관련한 다른 방식의 언급으로 시작한다: More than 25 years ago, a devastating form of immunodeficiency appeared, the acquired immune deficiency syndrome, or AIDS.

쉬운 영어로 과학논문 쓰는 법

첫째판 1쇄 인쇄 2015년 9월 23일
첫째판 1쇄 발행 2015년 10월 5일

지 은 이 ANNE E. GREENE
옮 긴 이 안성민
발 행 인 장주연
출 판 기 획 변연주
내 지 디 자 인 심현정
표 지 디 자 인 김민경
발 행 처 군자출판사
　　　　　　　등록 제4-139호(1991.6.24)
　　　　　　　본사 (110-717) 서울시 종로구 창경궁로 117(인의동 112-1) 동원회관 BD 6층
　　　　　　　전화 (02)762-9194/9197　　　팩스 (02)764-0209
　　　　　　　홈페이지 | www.koonja.co.kr

· 파본은 교환하여 드립니다.
· 검인은 저자와 합의 하에 생략합니다.

ISBN 978-89-6278-029-1
정가 15,000원